Biliary Tract Cancers

Guest Editor

JOSEPH J. BENNETT, MD, FACS

SURGICAL ONCOLOGY CLINICS OF NORTH AMERICA

www.surgonc.theclinics.com

Consulting Editor
NICHOLAS J. PETRELLI, MD

April 2009 • Volume 18 • Number 2

SAUNDERS an imprint of ELSEVIER, Inc.

W.B. SAUNDERS COMPANY
A Division of Elsevier Inc.

1600 John F. Kennedy Boulevard • Suite 1800 • Philadelphia, PA 19103-2899

http://www.theclinics.com

SURGICAL ONCOLOGY CLINICS OF NORTH AMERICA Volume 18, Number 2
April 2009 ISSN 1055-3207, ISBN-13: 978-1-4377-0912-4, ISBN-10: 1-4377-0912-5

Editor: Catherine Bewick
Developmental Editor: Donald Mumford

Surgical Oncology Clinics of North America (ISSN 1055-3207) is published quarterly by Elsevier Inc., 360 Park Avenue South, New York, NY 10010-1710. Months of publication are January, April, July, and October. Business and editorial offices: 1600 John F. Kennedy Boulevard, Suite 1800, Philadelphia, PA 19103-2899. Customer service office: 11830 Westline Industrial Drive, St. Louis, MO 63146. Periodicals postage paid at New York, NY, and additional mailing offices. Subscription prices are $218.00 per year (US individuals), $333.00 (US institutions) $110.00 (US student/resident), $251.00 (Canadian individuals), $414.00 (Canadian institutions), $158.00 (Canadian student/resident), $314.00 (foreign individuals), $414.00 (foreign institutions), and $158.00 (foreign student/resident). Foreign air speed delivery is included in all *Clinics* subscription prices. All prices are subject to change without notice. POST-MASTER: Send address changes to *Surgical Oncology Clinics of North America*, Elsevier Journals Customer Service, 11830 Westline Industrial Drive, St. Louis, MO 63146. **Customer Service: 1-800-654-2452 (US). From outside the United States, call 314-453-7041. Fax: 314-453-5170. E-mail: JournalsCustomerService-usa@elsevier.com (for print support); JournalsOnlineSupport-usa@elsevier. com (for online support).**

Reprints. For copies of 100 or more, of articles in this publication, please contact the Commercial Reprints Department, Elsevier Inc., 360 Park Avenue South, New York, New York 10010-1710. Tel. 212-633-3813; Fax: 212-462-1935; E-mail: reprints@elsevier.com.

Surgical Oncology Clinics of North America is covered in *MEDLINE/PubMed (Index Medicus) and EMBASE/ Excerpta Medica, Current Contents/Clinical Medicine, and ISI/BIOMED.*

Contributors

CONSULTING EDITOR

NICHOLAS J. PETRELLI, MD
Bank of America Endowed Medical Director, Helen F. Graham Cancer Center at Christiana
Care Health System, Newark, Delaware; and Professor of Surgery, Thomas Jefferson
University, Philadelphia, Pennsylvania

GUEST EDITOR

JOSEPH J. BENNETT, MD, FACS
Assistant Professor of Surgery, Thomas Jefferson University, Philadelphia, Pennsylvania;
Surgical Oncology Attending, Christiana Care Hospital and Helen F. Graham Cancer
Center, Newark, Delaware

AUTHORS

EDDIE K. ABDALLA, MD
Associate Professor, Department of Surgical Oncology, The University of Texas M.D.
Anderson Cancer Center, Houston, Texas

GHASSAN K. ABOU-ALFA, MD
Assistant Attending, Section of Gastrointestinal Oncology, Memorial Sloan-Kettering
Cancer Center, New York; Assistant Professor Weill Medical College at Cornell University,
New York, New York

GLENN S. ANDREWS, MD
Radiology Resident, Department of Radiology, Christiana Care Health System, Newark,
Delaware

JOSEPH J. BENNETT, MD, FACS
Assistant Professor of Surgery, Thomas Jefferson University, Philadelphia, Pennsylvania;
Surgical Oncology Attending, Christiana Care Hospital and Helen F. Graham Cancer
Center, Newark, Delaware

KAI BICKENBACH, MD
Surgical Resident, Department of Surgery, University of Chicago Pritzker School
of Medicine, Chicago, Illinois

CHERIF BOUTROS, MD, MSc
Department of Hepatobiliary and Surgical Oncology, Roger Williams Medical Center,
Boston University School of Medicine, Providence, Rhode Island

RACHEL E. BROCK, MD
Radiology Resident, Department of Radiology, Christiana Care Health System, Newark,
Delaware

DARREN R. CARPIZO, MD, PhD
Assistant Professor of Surgery, Division of Surgery, UMDNJ-Robert Wood Johnson Medical School, The Cancer Institute of New Jersey, New Brunswick, New Jersey

BRYAN M. CLARY, MD
Department of Surgery, Duke University Medical Center, Durham, North Carolina

MICHAEL D'ANGELICA, MD
Associate Attending Surgeon, Department of Surgery, Memorial Sloan-Kettering Cancer Center, New York; Assistant Professor of Surgery, Weill Medical College of Cornell University, New York, New York

MICHAEL A. DIGNAZIO, MD
Division of Interventional Radiology, Christiana Care Health System, Newark, Delaware

AUSTIN DUFFY, MD
Gastrointestinal Oncology Fellow, Section of Gastrointestinal Oncology, Memorial Sloan-Kettering Cancer Center, New York, New York

DAVID S. EPSTEIN, MD
Division of Interventional Radiology, Christiana Care Health System, Newark, Delaware

N. JOSEPH ESPAT, MD, MS
Professor of Surgery, Department of Hepatobiliary and Surgical Oncology, Roger Williams Medical Center, Boston University School of Medicine, Providence, Rhode Island

MANDIP S. GAKHAL, MD
Radiologist, Department of Radiology, Christiana Care Health System, Newark, Delaware

EVA GALKA, MD
Surgical Oncology Fellow, Department of Surgery, University of Chicago Pritzker School of Medicine, Chicago, Illinois

MARK J. GARCIA, MD, FSIR
Division of Interventional Radiology, Christiana Care Health System, Newark, Delaware

VINAY K. GHEYI, MD
Radiologist, Department of Radiology, Christiana Care Health System, Newark, Delaware

GREGORY J. GORES, MD
Professor of Medicine and Physiology, Chair, Division of Gastroenterology and Hepatology, Mayo Clinic College of Medicine, Rochester, Minnesota

RAYMOND H. GREEN, DO
General Surgery Resident, Department of Surgery, Christiana Care Hospital, Newark, Delaware

JULIE K. HEIMBACH, MD
Assistant Professor of Surgery, Division of Transplantation Surgery, Mayo Clinic College of Medicine, Rochester, Minnesota

FIDEL DAVID HUITZIL-MELENDEZ, MD
Gastrointestinal Oncology Fellow, Section of Gastrointestinal Oncology, Memorial Sloan-Kettering Cancer Center, New York, New York

NORIHIRO KOKUDO, MD, PhD
Professor, Division of Hepato-Biliary-Pancreatic Surgery, Department of Surgery,
Graduate School of Medicine, University of Tokyo, Tokyo, Japan

DAVID C. MADOFF, MD
Associate Professor, Department of Diagnostic Radiology, The University of Texas M.D.
Anderson Cancer Center, Houston, Texas

MASATOSHI MAKUUCHI, MD, PhD
President, Department of Surgery, Japanese Red Cross Medical Center, Tokyo, Japan

DAVID M. NAGORNEY, MD
Professor of Surgery, Division of Gastrointestinal and General Surgery, Mayo Clinic
College of Medicine, Rochester, Minnesota

EILEEN M. O'REILLY, MD
Associate Attending, Section of Gastrointestinal Oncology, Memorial Sloan-Kettering
Cancer Center New York; Associate Professor, Weill Medical College at Cornell
University, New York, New York

MARTIN PALAVECINO, MD
Post-Doctoral Research Fellow, Department of Surgical Oncology, The University
of Texas M.D. Anderson Cancer Center, Houston, Texas

DAVID J. REA, MD
Instructor in Surgery and Fellow, Division of Transplantation Surgery, Mayo Clinic College
of Medicine, Rochester, Minnesota

SRINEVAS K. REDDY, MD
Department of Surgery, Duke University Medical Center, Durham, North Carolina

KEVIN KING ROGGIN, MD
Assistant Professor of Surgery and Cancer Research, Department of Surgery,
University of Chicago Pritzker School of Medicine, Chicago, Illinois

CHARLES B. ROSEN, MD
Professor of Surgery, Division of Transplantation Surgery, Mayo Clinic College
of Medicine, Rochester, Minnesota

YASUJI SEYAMA, MD, PhD
Assistant Professor, Division of Hepato-Biliary-Pancreatic Surgery, Department
of Surgery, Graduate School of Medicine, University of Tokyo, Tokyo, Japan

PONNANDAI SOMASUNDAR, MD
Department of Hepatobiliary and Surgical Oncology, Roger Williams Medical Center,
Boston University School of Medicine, Providence, Rhode Island

JEAN-NICOLAS VAUTHEY, MD
Professor, Chief, Liver Service, Department of Surgical Oncology, The University of Texas
M.D. Anderson Cancer Center, Houston, Texas

Contents

> The hepatobiliary surgeon must be as familiar with the nonmalignant processes that can affect the extrahepatic biliary tree as they are with the malignant causes. Subtleties in the patient's history, presentation, and imaging studies may prevent unnecessary extensive hepatobiliary resection. The focus of this article deals with the etiology of nonmalignant obstruction at the biliary bifurcation and hilum and the mid-bile duct. It does not focus on either choledocholithiasis or pancreatitis, the two most common causes of distal bile duct obstruction. Obstruction from pancreatic cancer is also not the focus of this discussion.

> Cholangiocarcinoma (CC) is a rare, malignant neoplasm that can develop from any site within the intrahepatic or extrahepatic biliary tree. Although the key steps of cholangiocarcinogenesis remain unknown, it has been hypothesized that CC may develop through two key premalignant precursor lesions: biliary intraepithelial neoplasia (BilIN) and intraductal papillary neoplasm of the bile duct (IPNB). These lesions probably are analogous to pancreatic intraepithelial neoplasia and intraductal papillary mucinous neoplasm, respectively. This article outlines the molecular basis of cholangiocarcinogenesis through the BilIN and IPNB pathways. It highlights the genetic mutations that alter cellular proliferation, tumor suppression, and impairment of critical mucinous, cell-adhesion, and matrix proteins.

> Detection, accurate staging, and optimal management of biliary malignancies continue to present a significant challenge. This article reviews the current capabilities and roles of the various imaging modalities available in clinical practice, followed by a discussion of their integrated use at initial presentation, particularly with respect to potential surgical management of central hilar and intrahepatic cholangiocarcinoma. The main imaging modalities include MRI, CT, ultrasound, positron emission tomography, and

intrahepatic cholangiocarcinoma. Treatment options in unresectable patients are also reviewed.

This article describes the epidemiology, risk factors, diagnostic imaging tools, and operative management of gallbladder cancer. The rarity of gallbladder cancer coupled with the prevalence of benign gallbladder disease mean that most patients undergo initial procedures that violate tumor planes, complicating attempts at future oncologic resection. Fortunately, a previous laparoscopic or open cholecystectomy does not lessen survival after definitive surgical extirpation. Large retrospective and underpowered prospective studies have suggested benefit to adjuvant chemotherapy or radiotherapy; however, these results need to be confirmed with large prospective randomized trials.

Liver transplantation for cholangiocarcinoma has historically been maligned. Because of a high recurrence rate and poor patient survival, the disease has been viewed as an absolute contraindication to transplantation. Based on good results using neoadjuvant and palliative radiation, a protocol for liver transplantation in selected patients with unresectable hilar cholangiocarcinoma was developed in 1993. Neoadjuvant radiation is followed by operative staging to rule out patients with lymph node metastases before liver transplantation. This approach has achieved results superior to standard surgical therapy, with 72% 5-year survival for patients with unresectable disease.

Extended hemihepatectomy and/or pancreatoduodenectomy plus extrahepatic bile duct resection and an extended lymphadenectomy of up to the group 2 lymph nodes can enable long-term survival in patients with extrahepatic bile duct (EBD) cancer with acceptable surgical risks. Surgeons should dissect and examine at least 10 or more nodes in curative intent surgeries for local disease control and accurate staging. Radical surgical procedures for EBD cancer, including a right lobectomy, left trisectoriectomy, hepatopancreatoduodenectomy, and combined vascular resection and reconstruction, are useful options for obtaining a negative margin, but the benefits of such procedures to long-term survival rates is limited to selected patients without nodal metastasis and with negative surgical margins.

> Advanced biliary tract carcinomas represent a group of aggressive diseases that still carries a poor prognosis. Chemotherapy has been shown to provide disease control and may also prolong survival. An established role for systemic therapy in the adjuvant setting is still lacking. This article reviews the available evidence to support indications of systemic chemotherapy in the palliative setting and discuss the attempts to study it in the perioperative settings.

THE CLINICS ARE NOW AVAILABLE ONLINE!

Access your subscription at:
www.theclinics.com

Foreword

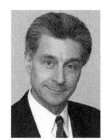

Nicholas J. Petrelli, MD
Consulting Editor

This issue of the *Surgical Oncology Clinics of North America* is devoted to biliary tract cancers. The Guest Editor is Joseph Bennett, MD, FACS. Dr. Bennett completed his general surgery training at the University of Chicago, which was subsequently followed by a surgical oncology fellowship at Memorial Sloan-Kettering Cancer Center. He presently is the Co-Director of the Hepatobiliary-Pancreatic Multidisciplinary Center at the Helen F. Graham Cancer Center at Christiana Care, and Assistant Professor of Surgery at Thomas Jefferson University.

In the United States in 2008, there were approximately 21,000 people with liver and extrahepatic bile duct cancers. In addition, there were approximately 9,500 people with gallbladder and extrahepatic biliary cancers. One can divide biliary tract cancers into those of the gallbladder, the ampulla of Vater, the extrahepatic bile ducts and the intrahepatic bile ducts. Interestingly, cholangiocarcinoma originally described primary tumors of the intrahepatic bile ducts and not those located extrahepatically. However, in recent times, cholangiocarcinoma has included intrahepatic, perihilar and distal extrahepatic cancers of the bile ducts. In 1965, Klatskin described perihilar tumors involving the bifurcation of the hepatic duct which today bears his name.

Like the overwhelming majority of tumors in the digestive system, biliary tract cancers are predominantly carcinomas. The most common histologic types are adenocarcinoma, mucinous and papillary carcinoma. Interestingly, because of the severe desmoplastic reaction of cholangiocarcinomas, it makes it difficult, especially in patients with cholangitis or intraductal gallstones, to distinguish between fibrous tissue and well differentiated cholangiocarcinoma. These issues and many others are described by Dr. Bennett and the expert group of physicians that he has put together for this issue of *Surgical Oncology Clinics of North America*. Dr. Bennett's own chapter, "Malignant Masquerade: Dilemmas in Diagnosing Biliary Obstruction" is must reading for surgical residents and fellows. Also, Dr. Kai Bickenbach from the University of Chicago discusses the molecular mechanisms of cholangiocarcinogenesis. In addition, there is an excellent discussion by our colleagues from M.D. Anderson Cancer Center on portal vein embolization and hilar cholangiocarcinoma.

Surg Oncol Clin N Am 18 (2009) xiii–xiv
doi:10.1016/j.soc.2009.02.002
surgonc.theclinics.com
1055-3207/09/$ – see front matter © 2009 Elsevier Inc. All rights reserved.

I want to congratulate Dr. Bennett and his colleagues for an outstanding issue of *Surgical Oncology Clinics of North America*. I look forward to sharing this edition with our own surgical residents at the Helen F. Graham Cancer Center.

Nicholas J. Petrelli, MD
Helen F. Graham Cancer Center
4701 Ogletown-Stanton Road
Suite 1213
Newark, DE 19713, USA

Department of Surgery
Jefferson Medical College
Philadelphia, PA 19107, USA

E-mail address:
npetrelli@christianacare.org

Preface

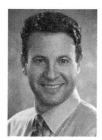

Joseph J. Bennett, MD, FACS
Guest Editor

The treatment of bile duct cancers has evolved tremendously in the last few decades. In 1983, Dr. Leslie Blumgart presented his experience on resecting hilar cholangiocarcinomas at the Southern Surgical Association, demonstrating a survival benefit when compared to palliative bypass.[1] The manuscript was met with criticism from other hepatobiliary surgeons and readers were cautioned about the data being presented, which stated that there is a difference between what "can be done" and what "should be done." One prominent surgeon said that he did not find any value to "curative" resection for bile duct cancers, noting that such efforts are futile. Such extensive operations only treat "the surgeon's capacity or need for rationalization," and allow the surgeon "to treat him- or herself for justification of self instead of treating the patient."

Yet here we are a quarter of a century later, and the pioneering work and perseverance of many surgeons, despite the nay sayers, have continued to improve patient quality and quantity of life, have expanded the indications and possibilities for extensive hepatic resection, and have made operations for bile duct malignancies much safer to perform. The articles included in this issue demonstrate what progress has been made since the last edition was published, not only in the field of surgery, but also in regards to radiology and body imaging, interventional radiology, novel chemotherapy regimens and finally, a better understanding of the cellular and molecular mechanisms that will need to be attacked to ultimately cure this disease. These articles have been written by nationally and internationally known authors and busy practicing physicians, and I certainly thank them for taking the time to contribute to this issue.

Treating bile duct malignancies requires surgeons to think outside the box and to push the limits, which is what attracts many of us to the field of hepatobiliary surgery in the first place. Hopefully such excitement is captured in this edition of *Surgical Oncology Clinics of North America*. The issue was designed to be comprehensive and if desired, to be read cover to cover to take the reader from initial diagnosis to imaging, percutaneous drainage and treatment, through the surgical options for the different types of biliary tract cancers, and then to adjuvant treatments and future molecular therapies. Each article also clearly stands by itself as a comprehensive update on the subject. As you read through these chapters keep in mind that what "can be done" soon becomes what "should be done," and what now seems radical may very well pave the road to a new future.

Surg Oncol Clin N Am 18 (2009) xv–xvi
doi:10.1016/j.soc.2009.02.001
surgonc.theclinics.com

Finally, I would like to thank Dr. Nicholas Petrelli for recruiting me to the Helen F. Graham Cancer Center, and for providing me with amazing opportunities for both personal and professional growth. I have had the privilege of being part of his creation, making a National Cancer Institute designated cancer center within a large community hospital, capable of treating any type of cancer and with the same level of expertise that's found at any university program. He has shown me that if you bring the right people together you can accomplish anything.

Joseph J. Bennett, MD, FACS
Helen F. Graham Cancer Center
4701 Ogletown-Stanton Road
Suite 1205 B
Newark, DE 19713, USA

E-mail address:
jobennett@christianacare.org (J.J. Bennett)

REFERENCE

1. Beazley RM, Hadjis N, Benjamin IS, et al. Clinicopathological aspects of high bile duct cancer: experience with resection and bypass surgical treatments. Ann Surg 1984;199(6):623–34.

Malignant Masquerade: Dilemmas in Diagnosing Biliary Obstruction

Joseph J. Bennett, MD, FACS[a,b,c,*], Raymond H. Green, DO[c]

KEYWORDS

- Malignant masquerade • Cholangiocarcinoma
- Benign biliary stricture

Cholangiocarcinoma is a challenging disease to treat, with most of the literature focusing on surgical resection, novel imaging modalities, adjuvant therapy, and palliative therapy. Much of the difficulty in treating extrahepatic biliary cancers actually begins, however, with the simple yet complex problem of just establishing a tissue diagnosis. It is paramount that the hepatobiliary surgeon is just as familiar with the nonmalignant processes that can affect the extrahepatic biliary tree as they are with the malignant causes. Subtleties in the patient's history, presentation, and imaging studies may prevent unnecessary extensive hepatobiliary resection. Although such resections have become safer and more commonplace at tertiary referral centers over the past few decades, it should not be taken for granted that such operations are still associated with a 30% to 50% morbidity and a 5% mortality. Missing the diagnosis of a malignancy, however, is a fatal mistake. This article deals with the etiology of nonmalignant obstruction at the biliary bifurcation and hilum and the mid-bile duct, and does not focus on either choledocholithiasis or pancreatitis, the two most common causes of distal bile duct obstruction. Obstruction from pancreatic cancer is also not the focus of this discussion.

DEFINITION

Nonmalignant causes of biliary obstruction are inflammatory processes creating diagnostic problems in that they frequently resemble malignancy. Hadjis and associates[1] coined the phrase "malignant masquerade" to describe these nonmalignant processes, further defined by Corvera and colleagues[2] as fibroinflammatory processes at the hilum

[a] Department of Surgical Oncology, Thomas Jefferson University, Philadelphia, PA, USA
[b] Helen F. Graham Cancer Center, 4701 Ogletown-Stanton Road, Suite 1205B, Newark, DE 19713, USA
[c] Department of Surgery, Christiana Care Hospital, 4755 Ogletown-Stanton Road, Newark, DE 19718, USA
* Corresponding author. Christiana Care Hospital and Helen F. Graham Cancer Center, 4701 Ogletown-Stanton Road, Newark, DE 19713, USA.
E-mail address: jobennett@christianacare.org (J.J. Bennett).

Surg Oncol Clin N Am 18 (2009) 207–214
doi:10.1016/j.soc.2008.12.005
1055-3207/08/$ – see front matter © 2009 Elsevier Inc. All rights reserved.

surgonc.theclinics.com

of the liver that are clinically indistinguishable from hilar cholangiocarcinoma. The number of patients found to possess a masquerade on final pathology is a minority when compared with those with a final diagnosis of cancer; however, numerous reports demonstrate the incidence of benign biliary stricture approaches 15%.[3] Because of the generic inflammatory process of the masquerade there have been many different causes elucidated in the literature over the last 20 years, some as simple as Mirizzi's syndrome, and others as obscure as a stricture of the bile duct caused by injection of a sclerosant performed as treatment for a bleeding duodenal ulcer.[4]

In differentiating benign biliary stricture from cholangiocarcinoma, radiologic studies have not been as helpful as one would suspect. Quite often patients who present with the clinical suspicion of biliary duct obstruction undergo a series of radiographic evaluations, including but not limited to CT scan, percutaneous transhepatic cholangiography (PTC), endoscopic retrograde cholangiopancreatography (ERCP), and positron emission tomography (PET). Although these tests have patterns that are suggestive of malignancy, none can obtain the specificity that can accurately differentiate between a benign stricture versus cholangiocarcinoma. Unfortunately, a large amount of the data present in the literature over the past 30 years concerning the conundrum between benign stricture and cholangiocarcinoma has not been statistically strong. Many of the early papers were centered on case reports and a few small series, all of which were inconclusive in making recommendations to help differentiate benign and malignant disease.

SEROLOGIC STUDIES

Serologic evaluations and the search for a tumor marker have historically come up short when differentiating benign from malignant stricture. Several tests have been studied including standard liver function testing, biliary fibronectin,[5] carcinoembryonic antigen, and CA 19-9.[6] CA 19-9 has been reported to be elevated in up to 85% of patients with cholangiocarcinoma; however, there are several studies to show that other benign processes can also cause CA 19-9 elevation.[6] CA 19-9 cannot discriminate between pancreatic malignancy, gastric malignancy, or cholangiocarcinoma and has also been shown to be elevated in primary sclerosing cholangitis (PSC). In a study by Safi and colleagues,[7] CA 19-9 was found to be elevated in 44% of patients with benign jaundice, and the elevated bilirubin itself was not found to alter the sensitivity of CA 19-9, indicating the true limitations of this test in differentiating between benign and malignant processes. Carcinoembryonic antigen has also been shown to be elevated in approximately 40% to 50% of patients with cholangiocarcinoma, but can also be elevated in more benign processes, such as inflammatory bowel disease and severe liver injury. Many other markers including, but not limited to, CA-125, CA-195, CA-242, DU-PAN-2, interleukin-6, and trypsinogen-2, have been tested but their clinical application has not yet been elucidated. Again, although there are patterns to suggest malignancy over benign stricture, the serologic tests all lack the specificity accurately to predict benign versus malignant cause for the disease process.

RADIOGRAPHIC EVALUATION OF CHOLANGIOCARCINOMA

When discussing the diagnostic evaluation for patients with suspected cholangiocarcinoma, a radiographic evaluation is certain. The question of which radiographic tests can assist in the diagnosis of biliary obstruction is not as difficult as discerning which radiographic test differentiates malignant from benign. It is accepted that almost all patients who present with biliary obstruction will most certainly undergo ultrasonographic evaluation of the biliary tree. Ultrasound (US) can assist with the diagnosis of biliary obstruction, and when intrahepatic ductal dilation in the absence of extrahepatic ductal dilation is present, a high suspicion for proximal cholangiocarcinoma may arise. Unfortunately, the sensitivity and specificity of US in differentiating benign versus malignant is poor. US is useful in that it is portable, widely available, and noninvasive. It can also be helpful for eliminating stone disease as a possible cause of biliary stricture, although the presence of cholelithiasis does not necessarily exclude the possibility that a cholangiocarcinoma is present concomitantly. The downside to US lies in the fact that it is operator dependant with a wide range in sensitivity based on the examiner's skill level. Garber and coworkers[8] found that the sensitivity for defining a mass in the biliary tree is as low as 21% to 47%. Despite this dismal sensitivity for identifying a mass, the study went on to report that US, based on tumor appearance and tumor mapping, has a high positive predictive value for diagnosing cholangiocarcinoma and is accurate in describing tumor site and extent of locoregional invasion. They found positive predictive values of 94% (verified by cholangiography in 78% of the patients), and were also able to identify extensive regional lymphadenopathy, liver lesions, and portal vein invasion, all of which are associated with malignant disease and much less likely with benign strictures. It should be strongly noted, however, that liver abscesses can appear like metastatic disease, adenopathy is not specific to malignancy, and even portal vein thrombosis has been seen in patients with benign inflammatory processes. In an evaluation of 171 patients who presented to Memorial Sloan-Kettering Cancer Center with hilar obstruction, the presence of vascular invasion was strongly associated with a final diagnosis of cholangiocarcinoma as compared with benign disease.[9] The sensitivity of vascular invasion was highest when associated with lobar atrophy, which can also be seen on US, but which is very operator dependent.

CT is frequently a second-line radiographic evaluation in the diagnosis of biliary obstruction for patients found to lack stone disease on US. CT can be quite helpful for delineating the biliary system, both intrahepatic and extrahepatic, and gives tremendous information about the liver parenchyma, regional lymph nodes, vascular involvement, and can identify metastatic disease. In this issue of *Surgical Oncology Clinics of North America*, there is an article addressing the radiologic evaluation of cholangiocarcinomas. In regards to malignant masquerade, however, a retrospective study by Choi and coworkers[10] identified some findings that were observed more frequently in malignant strictures and may help differentiate this entity from benign biliary stricture: a stricture wall thicker than 1.5 mm; a longer involved segment of duct (17.9 mm ± 6.6 mm for malignancy, versus benign at 8.9 mm ± 6.8 mm [$P< 0.0001$]); and a more dilated duct proximal to the obstruction (22 mm ± 5.4 mm for malignancy, versus benign at 17.8 mm ± 4.6 mm [$P = 0.033$]). The study further demonstrated that a hyperenhancement pattern of the involved bile duct wall during the portal venous phase is the main feature distinguishing benign biliary strictures from malignant ones ($P < .0001$) and can be used as an independent predictor to differentiate these two entities. Although this study shows promise, subsequent follow-up needs to be performed.

CT is also excellent in identifying lymphadenopathy. Although both ductal dilation and lymphadenopathy are components of cholangiocarcinoma, they are not specific for the disease. Lymphadenopathy can be present in a host of inflammatory processes, such as PSC, and as mentioned with US, ductal dilation is a nonspecific finding of both benign and malignant biliary stricture. Perhaps most valuable, triple-phase CT scan can identify vascular invasion and assess the resulting atrophy-hypertrophy that can be associated with biliary obstruction. Are and coworkers[9] demonstrated that vascular invasion occurs much more frequently in patients with malignancy, 58% versus 16% for patients with benign disease. Lobar atrophy also was found in 41% of patients with malignancy as compared with only 6% of patients with benign biliary stricture. In their series of 171 total patients where nine patients (5%) had a final histologic diagnosis of benign biliary stricture, however, none of these patients had vascular involvement but one patient did have lobar atrophy, indicating that even these prognostic variables are not perfect in attempting to avoid resection for malignant masquerade.

Cholangiography is an important part of the evaluation of biliary stricture. It is used both for the diagnosis of biliary stricture and planning for the resection of a stricture or mass. There are several different ways of performing cholangiography: ERCP, magnetic resonance cholangiopancreatography (MRCP), or PTC. ERCP is a common choice and is frequently chosen over PTC because of the ease of its performance, availability, and because most patients with obstructive jaundice have either choledocholithiasis or a periampullary neoplasm, both of which are diagnosed or treated by ERCP. PTC is often used when ERCP is unable to be performed, and is preferred once the diagnosis of a proximal biliary obstruction is made, especially when surgery is being considered and the future liver remnant needs to be drained.

Historically, MRI-MRCP has been shown to have a high sensitivity in detecting biliary obstruction (72%–98%) but has not repeatedly been shown to be sensitive at differentiating benign from malignant disease, with a wide range of sensitivities in the literature (30%–98%).[11] Recently MRCP has been shown to be equivalent to both ERCP and PTC in the evaluation of benign versus malignant disease. The MRCP comparison comes from studies by Park and coworkers[11] and Rösch and coworkers[12] who compared MRCP with both ERCP and PTC. They compared radiographic evaluation of ERCP and PTC versus MRCP and found that based on limited criteria (mostly anatomic appearance), the three modalities were equivalent at determining benign versus malignant disease. Rösch and coworkers[12] did submit that although the sensitivity may be similar, both modalities lack specificity and that ERCP may provide a tissue diagnosis, relegating MRCP to a more limited clinical role. It is important to keep in mind that ERCP and biopsy does not often provide a tissue diagnosis either, especially for more proximal lesions. In regards to MRCP, when a malignant diagnosis is being considered, contrast-enhanced MRI should be ordered in conjunction with MRCP and provides excellent information regarding the liver parenchyma (including atrophy-hypertrophy, and evaluating for liver metastases), vascular invasion, and lymph node status, and provides similar or adjunctive data to CT scan.

When considering patients for radiographic evaluation for malignancy, PET scanning has been shown to be an effective method for identifying highly metabolically active areas consistent with tumor. It is logical to consider the use of PET in the evaluation of biliary stricture because PET has been shown in numerous studies to be useful for the diagnosis of cholangiocarcinoma.[13–18] There are some studies that have shown that PET in association with CT scanning (so-called "PET-CT") has allowed for a greater chance at curative resection secondary to their ability to evaluate regional lymphadenopathy and distant metastasis. This allowed for more accurate assessment of patients, upgrading some to unresectable and downgrading others to resectable disease versus only conventional imaging.[13] This meant curative resection for some, whereas sparing others from unwarranted laparotomy. When using PET scanning to evaluate a biliary stricture as benign versus malignant, however, PET falls short. PET currently lacks the sensitivity for diagnosing malignancy versus benign disease, especially mucinous cholangiocarcinoma, which lacks FDG avidity.

There has been some hope that PET may be useful for this determination in the near future.

TISSUE SAMPLING

In discussing the role of tissue sampling for benign biliary disease, it is important to realize that most biliary strictures (especially hilar stricture) in patients who have never undergone biliary tree manipulation, and who do not have stone disease, are ultimately adenocarcinoma. The collection of tissue for pathologic assessment has been used in the past mainly to obtain a positive tissue diagnosis so that the surgeon may begin operative planning. The converse is not, however, as clear cut. Obtaining tissue that is cytologically negative is more often a false-negative biopsy than a positive finding of benign biliary disease.[9] This is perhaps the most important point that an experienced hepatobiliary team needs to explain to a patient who is to undergo major resection but who has a negative biopsy. The most common ways to obtain tissue are either endoscopic US (EUS), PTC, or by ERCP. Previous studies demonstrate that the yield for brushings from ERCP or PTC have been positive in only 30% of patients with diagnosed cholangiocarcinoma.[9,19] In a recent prospective study Rösch and coworkers[20] compared EUS-guided fine-needle aspiration with ERCP brushings in 28 patients with biliary stricture who were later found to have a diagnosed malignancy. They showed that in patients who were ultimately diagnosed with a malignancy, the sensitivity was only 36% for ERCP with biopsy and 46% when brushings were performed. Patients were randomized during this study to the use of one of three different methods for tissue collection: (1) conventional over-the-guidewire cytology brush, (2) a spiral cytology brush, and (3) intrabiliary forceps. EUS-guided fine-needle aspiration specificity was not much better at 43%.[20] Some recent data show higher sensitivity and specificity with biliary brush cytology for the early (in situ) diagnosis of cholangiocarcinoma in PSC, with a sensitivity of 70% to 100% and specificity of 80% to 95%.[21]

CAUSES OF BENIGN BILIARY STRICTURE

When considering the causes of benign biliary stricture, there are a wide variety of reports in the literature. The pathologic causes can be grouped into five general categories, as described by Corvera and coworkers:[2] (1) lymphoplasmacytic sclerosing pancreatitis and cholangitis, (2) PSC, (3) nonspecific fibroinflammatory process, (4) granulomatous disease, and (5) stone disease.

Lymphoplasmacytic sclerosing pancreatitis and cholangitis, also known as primary inflammatory sclerosis of the pancreas, sclerosing pancreatitis, autoimmune sclerosing pancreatitis, duct destructive chronic pancreatitis, and sclerosing pancreaticocholangitis, is characterized by diffuse fibroinflammatory lymphoplasmacytic infiltrates that can involve both the pancreatic ducts and acinar parenchyma. Lymphoplasmacytic sclerosing pancreatitis and cholangitis frequently involves the head of the pancreas and the distal bile duct and has been known to form masses that can resemble malignancy. It is also not limited to just the distal duct, and should be considered in the differential diagnosis when also considering cholangiocarcinoma. It primarily affects middle-aged men, and is frequently amenable to steroid therapy.[22] As with other causes of malignant masquerade, the trick is in the diagnosis. When considering a diagnosis of lymphoplasmacytic sclerosing pancreatitis and cholangitis, testing for serum IgG4 levels is the best discriminating test to differentiate a malignant from a benign process. Because the test is so simple and may change management quite dramatically, it is reasonable to check IgG4 levels in any patient with a biliary stricture where a tissue diagnosis has not been established.[23,24] If IgG4 levels are significantly elevated, a short course of steroids often provides resolution of biliary obstruction symptoms, which is certainly not seen if the patient has a malignant stricture.

PSC is a chronic cholestatic liver disease of unknown etiology that has its peak incidence in the third and fourth decades of life. It has a strong association with inflammatory bowel disease, because some 70% to 80% of patients with PSC have concomitant inflammatory bowel disease. Unlike with malignant causes of jaundice, patients with PSC usually have a cyclical nature to their symptoms, both clinically and when measuring liver function tests. Also unlike patients with malignant biliary obstruction, patients with PSC usually have multiple sites of strictures, which affect both the intrahepatic and extrahepatic biliary tree. This classic pattern of alternating strictures and dilatations results in a beading appearance on cholangiography, which is a hallmark of PSC and should be recognized as a benign entity. Single dominant strictures can occur in PSC, however, and should not negate the diagnosis. It is also important to note that up to one third of patients with PSC may develop a cholangiocarcinoma in their lifetime, further complicating the ability to differentiate between a benign stricture and a malignancy. Patients who develop cholangiocarcinoma in a background of PSC usually have long-standing disease, and so once again, the past medical history should help with the diagnosis.

Finally, in considering the causes of benign biliary stricture a final category should be considered: iatrogenic-idiopathic-autoimmune. A detailed past medical history should help in the diagnosis of some of these etiologies of obstruction. Multiple reports in the literature have shown benign biliary stricture after injection of sclerosant for duodenal ulceration,[4] as a consequence of non-Hodgkin's lymphoma,[25] pyogenic cholangitis,[26] atherosclerosis,[27] and there is at least one report of an idiopathic benign biliary stricture that was ultimately related to a local cholangitis that was not PSC. Several autoimmune processes have also been shown to cause biliary stricture, such as systemic lupus erythematosus, Wegner's granulomatosis, and Sjögren's syndrome, all either with or without granulomatous formation.[2,28]

SUMMARY

Cholangiocarcinoma is a devastating disease and surgery is the only option for cure. The ability to establish a definitive tissue diagnosis preoperatively for patients who seem to have radiographically resectable disease is unfortunately low. Surgeons have become appropriately aggressive to recommend major hepatobiliary resection in patients with a high index of suspicion for biliary tract cancers. Even in patients with resectable disease, 5-year survival rates are still only 30% to 35%.[29] Analyses of patients who have undergone resection have demonstrated that 5% to 15% of suspected malignant disease was ultimately benign on final pathology. It is the hepatobiliary surgeon's responsibility to be familiar with the many causes of malignant masquerade and to reduce the incidence of unnecessary resection, while also being prudent to make sure that a true malignancy is not missed. Unfortunately, no tests have been able accurately to differentiate between benign and malignant disease. As discussed, there are no specific radiographic findings on US, CT, MRI-MRCP, ERCP, EUS, or PET scan reliably to define benign disease. There is no laboratory value that can accurately and dependably diagnose biliary obstruction caused by adenocarcinoma. Patients need to be counseled regarding the fact that their biliary stricture may well be benign.

With an improved awareness of the etiology of malignant masquerade, and with better diagnostic tools likely in the near future, the incidence of malignant masquerade will not disappear. On the contrary, the authors make the opposing argument that if benign disease were never resected then many cholangiocarcinomas would likely be underdiagnosed and undertreated. It is hoped that the incidence can approach a level that is lower than the 5% to 15% that is currently being reported.

REFERENCES

1. Hadjis NS, Collier NA, Blumgart LH. Malignant masquerade at the hilum of the liver. Br J Surg 1985;72:659–61.
2. Corvera CU, Blumgart LH, Darvishian F, et al. Clinical and pathologic features of proximal biliary strictures masquerading as hilar cholangiocarcinoma. J Am Coll Surg 2005;201:862–9.
3. Gerhards MF, Vos P, van Gulik TM, et al. Incidence of benign lesions in patients resected for suspicious hilar obstruction. Br J Surg 2001;88:48–51.
4. Luman W, Hudson N, Choudari CP, et al. Distal biliary stricture as a complication of sclerosant injection for bleeding duodenal ulcer. Gut 1994;35:1665–7.
5. Chen CY, Lin XZ, Tsao HC, et al. The value of biliary fibronectin for diagnosis of cholangiocarcinoma. Hepatogastroenterology 2003;50:924–7.
6. Murray MD, Burton FR, Di Bisceglie AM. Markedly elevated serum CA 19-9 levels in association with a benign biliary stricture due to primary sclerosing cholangitis. J Clin Gastroenterol 2007;41:115–7.
7. Safi F, Schlosser W, Kolb G, et al. Diagnostic value of CA 19-9 in patients with pancreatic cancer and nonspecific gastrointestinal symptoms. J Gastrointest Surg 1997;1:106–12.
8. Garber SJ, Donald JJ, Lees WR. Cholangiocarcinoma: ultrasound features and correlation of tumor position with survival. Abdom Imaging 1993;18:66–9.
9. Are C, Gonen M, D'Angelica M, et al. Differential diagnosis of proximal biliary obstruction. Surgery 2006;140:756–63.
10. Choi SH, Han JK, Lee JM, et al. Differentiating malignant from benign common bile duct stricture with multiphasic helical CT. Radiology 2005;236:178–83.
11. Park MS, Kim TK, Kim KW, et al. Differentiation of extrahepatic bile duct cholangiocarcinoma from benign stricture: findings at MRCP versus ERCP. Radiology 2004;233:234–40.
12. Rosch T, Meining A, Fruhmorgen S, et al. A prospective comparison of the diagnostic accuracy of ERCP, MRCP, CT, and EUS in biliary strictures. Gastrointest Endosc 2002;55:870–6.
13. Kim JY, Kim MH, Lee TY, et al. Clinical role of 18F-FDG PET-CT in suspected and potentially operable cholangiocarcinoma: a prospective study compared with conventional imaging. Am J Gastroenterol 2008;103:1145–51.
14. Anderson CD, Rice MH, Pinson CW, et al. Fluorodeoxyglucose PET imaging in the evaluation of gallbladder carcinoma and cholangiocarcinoma. J Gastrointest Surg 2004;8:90–7.
15. Fritscher-Ravens A, Bohuslavizki KH, Broering DC, et al. FDG PET in the diagnosis of hilar cholangiocarcinoma. Nucl Med Commun 2001;22:1277–85.
16. Kato T, Tsukamoto E, Kuge Y, et al. Clinical role of (18)F-FDG PET for initial staging of patients with extrahepatic bile duct cancer. Eur J Nucl Med Mol Imaging 2002;29:1047–54.
17. Kim YJ, Yun M, Lee WJ, et al. Usefulness of 18F-FDG PET in intrahepatic cholangiocarcinoma. Eur J Nucl Med Mol Imaging 2003;30:1467–72.

18. Kluge R, Schmidt F, Caca K, et al. Positron emission tomography with [(18)F]flu-oro-2-deoxy-D-glucose for diagnosis and staging of bile duct cancer. Hepatology 2001;33:1029–35.
19. Khan SA, Davidson BR, Goldin R, et al. Guidelines for the diagnosis and treatment of cholangiocarcinoma: consensus document. Gut 2002;51(Suppl 6):vi1–9.
20. Rosch T, Hofrichter K, Frimberger E, et al. ERCP or EUS for tissue diagnosis of biliary strictures? A prospective comparative study. Gastrointest Endosc 2004; 60:390–6.
21. Boberg KM, Jebsen P, Clausen OP, et al. Diagnostic benefit of biliary brush cytology in cholangiocarcinoma in primary sclerosing cholangitis. J Hepatol 2006;45:568–74.
22. Kawamoto S, Siegelman SS, Hruban RH, et al. Lymphoplasmacytic sclerosing pancreatitis with obstructive jaundice: CT and pathology features. AJR Am J Roentgenol 2004;183:915–21.
23. Finkelberg DL, Sahani D, Deshpande V, et al. Autoimmune pancreatitis. N Engl J Med 2006;355:2670–6.
24. Hamano H, Kawa S, Horiuchi A, et al. High serum IgG4 concentrations in patients with sclerosing pancreatitis. N Engl J Med 2001;344:732–8.
25. Ravindra KV, Stringer MD, Prasad KR, et al. Non-Hodgkin lymphoma presenting with obstructive jaundice. Br J Surg 2003;90:845–9.
26. Yoon HK, Sung KB, Song HY, et al. Benign biliary strictures associated with recurrent pyogenic cholangitis: treatment with expandable metallic stents. AJR Am J Roentgenol 1997;169:1523–7.
27. Saiura A, Umekita N, Inoue S, et al. Benign biliary stricture associated with atherosclerosis. Hepatogastroenterology 2001;48:81–2.
28. Binkley CE, Eckhauser FE, Colletti LM. Unusual causes of benign biliary strictures with cholangiographic features of cholangiocarcinoma. J Gastrointest Surg 2002; 6:676–81.
29. Jarnagin WR, Fong Y, DeMatteo RP, et al. Staging, resectability, and outcome in 225 patients with hilar cholangiocarcinoma. Ann Surg 2001;234:507–17 [discussion: 517–9].

Molecular Mechanisms of Cholangiocarcinogenesis: Are Biliary Intraepithelial Neoplasia and Intraductal Papillary Neoplasms of the Bile Duct Precursors to Cholangiocarcinoma?

Kai Bickenbach, MD[1], Eva Galka, MD[1], Kevin King Roggin, MD*

KEYWORDS

- Cholangiocarcinoma • Biliary intraepithelial neoplasia
- Intraductal papillary neoplasm of the bile duct
- Molecular mechanisms of cholangiocarcinoma

Cholangiocarcinoma (CC) is a rare, malignant neoplasm that can develop from any site within the intrahepatic or extrahepatic biliary tree. Most occur at the hilum (50%) and within the extrahepatic bile ducts (42%); only 8% of these tumors originate in the intrahepatic biliary ducts (ie, intrahepatic CC or peripheral CC).[1] At the time of diagnosis, most CCs are unresectable. This delay in diagnosis has been attributed in part to the rarity of this disease in the United States population, the lack of specific symptoms, and the relative proximity of these tumors to critical structures. Long-term survival is possible only with complete surgical resection. Resectability rates are highest for extrahepatic CC and decrease with more proximal locations in the biliary tree (ie, in the hilum and peripheral bile ducts). Chemotherapy and radiation therapy are ineffective, noncurative treatments.[2] Improvements in long-term survival probably will parallel an increased understanding of the mechanisms of malignant transformation of biliary epithelium into CC.

Although the exact cause of CC remains unknown, most cited risk factors share several common features—infection, inflammation, cholestasis, and increased cholangiocyte turnover. Biliary tract malignancies have been associated with unresected

Department of Surgery, University of Chicago Pritzker School of Medicine, 5841 S Maryland Avenue, MC 6040, Chicago, IL 60637, USA
[1] Drs. Bickenbach and Galka share joint first authorship.
* Corresponding author.
E-mail address: kroggin@surgery.bsd.uchicago.edu (K.K. Roggin).

Surg Oncol Clin N Am 18 (2009) 215–224
doi:10.1016/j.soc.2008.12.001
1055-3207/08/$ – see front matter © 2009 Elsevier Inc. All rights reserved.

choledochal cystic disease, primary sclerosing cholangitis, hepatolithiasis, radiation exposure, previous biliary tract procedures or operations, viral infections (hepatitis and HIV), liver fluke infestation with *Opisthorchis viverrini* and *Clonorchis sinensis*, and exposure to carcinogens such as Thorotrast. These chronic injurious stimuli may transform normal epithelial cells into malignant lesions. Most epithelial cancers develop in a stepwise progression from normal mucosal cells to adenomatous hyperplasia, dysplasia, carcinoma in situ, and eventually an invasive cancer. This process is characterized by the acquisition of increasing mutations and molecular alterations stemming from DNA damage, alteration of the cell cycle regulators, and/or the sustained unregulated production of cytokines, growth factors, and hormones. This sequence of cancer development has been well characterized in colon, breast, and esophageal adenocarcinomas.[3–6] Although the key steps of cholangiocarcinogenesis remain unknown, it has been hypothesized that CC may develop through two key premalignant precursor lesions: biliary intraepithelial neoplasia (BilIN) and intraductal papillary neoplasm of the bile duct (IPNB). These lesions probably are analogous to pancreatic intraepithelial neoplasia (PanIN) and intraductal papillary mucinous neoplasm (IPMN), respectively. This article outlines the molecular basis of cholangiocarcinogenesis through the BilIN and IPNB pathways. It highlights genetic mutations that alter cellular proliferation, tumor suppression, and impairment of critical mucinous, cell-adhesion, and matrix proteins.

BILIARY INTRAEPITHELIAL NEOPLASIA

BilIN is characterized by a flat or micropapillary growth of atypical biliary epithelium. It previously was called "atypical biliary epithelia" and "biliary dysplasia." BilIN is characteristically a microscopic lesion that can progress to tubular adenocarcinoma. These premalignant lesions are classified commonly into three grades based on the degree of cellular and structural atypia: BilIN-1, BilIN-2, and BilIN-3.[7,8]

BilIN typically is found in large intrahepatic biliary ducts and rarely is present in septal or interlobular ducts. It is associated with conditions that cause chronic inflammation, including hepatolithiasis, choledochal cystic disease, liver fluke infestation, and primary sclerosing cholangitis. Liver fluke infestation and primary sclerosing cholangitis usually are associated with BilIN, not with IPNB lesions.

INTRADUCTAL PAPILLARY NEOPLASM OF THE BILE DUCT

IPNB is a macroscopic lesion characterized by prominent papillary growth of atypical biliary epithelium with a fibrovascular core and overproduction of mucin.[9] IPNB, like BilIN, occurs in bile ducts associated with chronic inflammatory conditions such as hepatolithiasis or choledochocysts. IPNB can transform into two types of invasive cancers, each with different biologic behavior and prognosis: mucinous carcinoma or tubular adenocarcinoma.[10] The histologic subtype of the invasive cancers developing within IPNB lesions seems to influence survival after resection. Survival rates in patients who have mucinous carcinoma are considerably better than in patients who have tubular adenocarcinoma.[11] Furthermore, IPNB-associated CC has a more favorable outcome than CC that develops through the BilIN pathways.[8,12] Once tubular adenocarcinoma develops from IPNB lesions, however, the reported survival rates are similar to those for nonpapillary CC and are worse than those for mucinous biliary cancers.[11] Nakanishi and colleagues[10] categorized IPNB into IPNB-1 (premalignant and borderline cases) and IPNB-2 (carcinoma in situ) using the World Health Organization criteria for pancreatic IPMN.

CELL-CYCLE PROTEINS

Cyclin D1 is a proto-oncogene that is an important regulator of cell-cycle progression from the G1 to S phase. The cyclin D1 protein forms a complex with cyclin-dependent kinase-4 and -6 (CDK4 and CDK6) that allows cells to progress into S phase by phosphorylation and inactivation of the retinoblastoma protein.[13] *Cyclin D1* is overexpressed in many cancers, including intrahepatic CC, a consequence of gene amplification or defective regulation at the posttranscriptional level.[14–16] *Cyclin D1* also binds to cyclin-dependent kinase-2 (CDK2) and CDK4 to promote cell-cycle progression and cellular proliferation. Overexpression of *cyclin D1* has been reported in as many as two thirds of patients who have intrahepatic CC and is associated with more biologically aggressive tumors with poor differentiation and lymph node metastasis.[15,17] Nakanishi and colleagues[10] demonstrated that abnormal *cyclin D1* levels parallel the histologic progression from BilIN-1 through BilIN-3 and eventually CC in resected specimens. This finding was confirmed in IPNB lesions, as well, by both Nakanishi and colleagues[10] and Itatsu and colleagues.[18] This paradigm seems to mirror the molecular progression of PanIN and IPMN to invasive cancer in pancreatic carcinogenesis.[19] In the study by Itatsu and colleagues,[18] expression of *cyclin D1* was more common in IPNB lesions (65%) than in BilIN lesions (20%), indicating that up-regulation of *cyclin D1* expression may be more important to the IPNB lineage. The Nakanishi[10] study, however, showed that there was no difference in expression between IPNB and BilIN lesions. More importantly, in both studies this difference in *cyclin D1* expression was lost when the invasive phenotype of either BilIN or IPNB was observed.[10,18] Thus, *cyclin D1* overexpression may represent a common pathway that transforms atypical cholangiocytes into CC in both BilIN and IPNB lesions.

Like *cyclin D1*, *p21* is a cyclin-dependent kinase inhibitor that prevents cell-cycle progression at the G1-S checkpoint. In normal cells, *p53* up-regulates *p21* to inhibit cell proliferation.[20] Nakanishi and colleagues[10] demonstrated that *p21* expression was increased significantly with progression to BilIN-2 and gradually was amplified in resected specimens. In the IPNB lineage, *p21* expression increased with histologic progression from IPNB-1 to IPNB-2 and was greatest in invasive CC specimens with IPNB features.[10] This finding suggests that overexpression of *p21* may be an early mechanism of cholangiocarcinogenesis in both the BilIN and IPNB pathways. Altered regulation of both *cyclin D1* and *p21* may lead to uncontrolled cellular proliferation, leading to increasing cholangiocyte atypia and eventually CC along both the BilIN and IPNB pathways.[19]

TUMOR SUPPRESSOR GENES

DPC4 (Smad4) is a tumor suppressor gene located on chromosome 18q and is a member of a highly conserved family of proteins involved in the transduction of signals from the transforming growth factor beta (TGF-β) family.[21] *DPC4* has been implicated in carcinogenesis through transmission of TGF-β epithelial growth inhibition signals.[21] *DPC4* mutations have been demonstrated in several reports of CC. Hahn and colleagues[22] showed that 16% of resected biliary tract cancers had a mutation in the *DPC4* gene. The loss of *DPC4* expression is more frequent in extrahepatic CC (55%) than in either hilar (15%) or intrahepatic CC (13%).[23] Immunohistochemistry staining confirmed that cellular *DPC4* expression gradually decreases with progression from both BilIN and IPNB into invasive CC in patient samples.[10] This pattern mirrors the loss of *DPC4* expression in the transformation of PanIN into invasive pancreatic cancers.[24]

Alterations of the *p53* tumor suppressor gene are the most common genetic mutations found in human cancers and result in uncontrolled cellular proliferation. The p53 gene product normally functions by initiating DNA repair, halts cell-cycle progression, and induces apoptosis. Altered metabolism of the mutated p53 product increases the intracellular levels of *p53*. Up-regulation of *p53* expression, therefore, is a surrogate marker for *p53* mutations. Overexpression of the mutated protein product has been identified in more than half of intrahepatic CC specimens and in as many as 80% of extrahepatic CC in selected series.[23,25–30] *p53* mutations detected by DNA sequencing have been identified in as many as one third of intrahepatic and extrahepatic CC.[25] Up-regulation of *p53* expression correlates with progressive premalignant BilIN.[10] *p53* overexpression has been identified in 11% of BilIN-3 and in 75% of invasive CC arising from BilIN lesions, but it rarely is identified in normal cholangiocytes, BilIN-1, or BilIN-2 lesions.[10] In contrast to the pattern in the BilIN lineage, up-regulation of *p53* expression was identified early in low-grade IPNB-1 lesions but was not increased further in IPNB-2 or IPNB-induced CC. These data suggest that *p53* mutations may be important in the advancement of BilIN lesions and may represent the acquisition of an invasive phenotype. These mutations seem to be less critical in the progression of IPNB lesions.[10] Instead, *p53* mutations may contribute to the initial development of IPNB lesions.

C-myc is a transcription factor that induces cellular growth and proliferation. It inhibits cellular apoptosis and is a target molecule of the Wnt signaling pathway.[18] C-myc overexpression has been identified in 10% to 41% of CC resected specimens.[31,32] Itatsu and colleagues[18] demonstrated low levels of c-myc expression in BilIN-1 (17%), BilIN-2 (18), and CC with BilIN (11%). In contrast, c-myc expression was up-regulated in more than half the IPNB lesions. C-myc expression was not identified in non-neoplastic biliary epithelium.[18] The expression of c-myc correlated with decreased membranous expression of *E-cadherin* and β-catenin in the IPNB lineage. This finding suggests that c-myc may not play an important role in development along the BilIN pathway but is more important in development of the IPNB pathway.

MUCINOUS PROTEINS

Mucin core proteins (MUC) are members of the mucin protein family that encode organ-specific glycoproteins produced by many epithelial tissues.[33] MUC are anti-adhesion molecules that, when altered, may facilitate cancer cell invasion through the basement membranes.[34,35] These proteins disrupt the normal adhesive interactions between cellular integrins and the extracellular matrix.[36,37] Abnormal levels of sialylated MUC1 protein have been demonstrated in many adenocarcinomas, including invasive CC. MUC1 has been associated with advanced tumors with poor differentiation, deep invasion, and lymphatic or perineural invasion.[33,36] The MUC2 protein product produces an intestinal-type secretory mucin that forms a protective mucous barrier in the gastrointestinal tract lumen. MUC2 expression has been identified in CC with more favorable biologic phenotypes (ie, well-differentiated CC and noninvasive cancers).[12,38] Normal intrahepatic bile ducts and nonpapillary CC do not express MUC2.

MUC1 is present in up to one quarter of all BilIN and has been seen in the majority of resected CC that develop through BilIN precursor lesions.[10,11] This finding suggests that the MUC1 overexpression is a key, late step in the transformation of BilIN into CC. MUC2 expression does not seem to be critical to the BilIN cholangiocarcinogenesis; it is seen in only 13.2% to 21% of BilIN tumors and in 9.1% to 17% of CC with

BilIN. This pattern of MUC1 and MUC2 expression parallels the findings reported in PanIN-induced pancreatic adenocarcinomas.[39]

Yonezawa and Sato[33] found that MUC1 was highly expressed in invasive CC but rarely was identified in IPNB with CC. Likewise, Nakanishi and colleagues[10] reported that MUC1 expression was seen less commonly in resected IPNB lesions; only 12.5% of IPNB lesions and 60% of CC that developed from IPNB precursor lesions expressed MUC1. MUC1-positive lesions commonly develop into tubular adenocarcinoma, and IPNB lesions without MUC1 expression are associated more frequently with mucinous carcinoma.[11] It seems that MUC1 proteins regulate the differentiation of IPNB into either tubular adenocarcinoma or mucinous carcinoma. Several studies found that MUC2 expression parallels the progression of IPNB lesions.[9] Survival rates seem to be better in patients who have MUC2-positive tumors than in patients who have MUC2-negative tumors.[40] It is possible that MUC2 expression facilitates the growth of tumors with a decreased capacity for invasion and metastasis.[33]

CELL-ADHESION PROTEINS

Alterations in normal cell-adhesion molecules may be an important determinant of cancer invasion and metastatic potential. *E-cadherin* is a tumor suppressor gene that produces a transmembrane protein involved in epithelial cell adhesion.[41] The extracellular domain functions through calcium-dependent, homophilic interactions with the extracellular matrix. The intracellular portion is a catenin-like protein that transmits signals related to cell adhesion. Reduced expression of *E-cadherin* and/or mutations in the gene may foster increased invasiveness and loss of cellular differentiation. As lesions progress from premalignant to the invasive phenotype, *E-cadherin* often is suppressed or altered. Decreased expression and mutations of *E-cadherin* have been reported in CC and are associated with poorly differentiated tumors. Although *E-cadherin* expression often is preserved in non-neoplastic biliary epithelium, the gene is muted or altered with progression of both BilIN and IPNB lesions. Although *E-cadherin* expression was decreased only slightly in BilIN-1 -2, and -3 (compared with non-neoplastic epithelium), it was suppressed significantly in CC that developed from BilIN and IPNB lesions.[18] This finding suggests that loss of *E-cadherin* function may be a late change in the development of the invasive phenotype in both BilIN and IPNB.

β-catenin is a cytoplasmic protein that is intimately associated with the cadherin family. These proteins mediate cell adhesion and act as downstream signaling mediators of the wingless-Wnt signal transduction pathway. Reduced expression of β-catenin at the cytoplasmic cell membrane is thought to disrupt cell adhesion and promote invasion.[42] Nuclear translocation of β-catenin can contribute to carcinogenesis through activation of c-myc, *cyclin D1*, and matrix metalloproteinase (MMP)-7 transcription.[42–44] Decreased β-catenin has been reported in multiple tumors, including CC.[45] Studies have demonstrated that 58% to 82% of CC have decreased membrane expression of β-catenin.[46] Itatsu and colleagues[18] showed that membranous expression of β-catenin in resected specimens gradually decreased with progression from BilIN-1 to BilIN-3 and was lowest in CC arising from BilIN lesions. Likewise, β-catenin expression was decreased with progression of IPNB lesions and was decreased significantly with CC with IPNB. This finding suggests that loss of cell-adhesion properties mediated by β-catenin and *E-cadherin* are important steps in cholangiocarcinogenesis through both premalignant pathways. Nuclear staining of β-catenin, however, was found only in the IPNB lineage (22%) and probably reflects the activation of the Wnt signaling pathway.[18]

MATRIX PROTEINS

MMPs are critical proteins that metabolize extracellular matrix. Their physiologic activity is a complex dynamic between MMP activity, MMP inhibitors (ie, TIMP-1, TIMP-2), and the extracellular milieu (ie, electrolytes, stroma, and other chemical mediators). Overexpression of MMP may promote epithelial cancer invasion and metastasis. Several studies have demonstrated an increased expression of membrane-type metalloproteinase-1 (MT1)-MMP and MMP-7 in resected CC.[47,48] MT1-MMP degrades type 1 collagen and extracellular adhesion molecules. It also disrupts the normal mitotic spindle that is critical to chromosomal alignment and distribution during mitosis.[39,40] Daughter-cell DNA aneuploidy may facilitate malignant transformation of cholangiocytes.[49,50] MMP-7 degrades extracellular collagens, proteoglycans, lamins, and fibronectin. Overexpression of both MMP-7 and MT1-MMP has been demonstrated in CC and is associated with a poor histologic grade and prognosis.[47]

Although MT1-MMP and MMP-7 expression were not present in early BilIN lesions, they were expressed consistently in late BilIN lesions (BilIN-2 and -3) and in all BilIN-associated CC in resected samples.[18] This finding suggests that changes in MMP may be a late occurrence as BilIN progresses to an invasive phenotype. Expression of MMP-7 in resected IPNB lesions was low (10%) compared with BilIN lesions.[18] This difference may contribute to the less invasive phenotype of IPNB lesions as compared with BilIN lesions.

SUMMARY

Two key premalignant lesions, BilIN and IPNB, have been implicated in the development of CC. These tumors share similarities with their pancreatic analogues, PanIN and IPMN. Each of these lesions follows different tumorigenic pathways with distinct genetic alterations (**Table 1**). Lesions of the BilIN and PanIN lineage develop a gradual progression of mutations in *cyclin D1*, *p21*, and *p53* with greater loss of *DPC4* and molecular cell adhesion expression. BilIN lesions have significantly higher expression of MMP-7 and MT1-MMP than their IPNB counterparts, corresponding to the greater

Table 1
Immunohistochemical expression of cell-cycle proteins, mucin core proteins, and matrix metalloproteinases in BilIN and IPNB lesions

Entity	Cyclin D1	p21	p53	DPC4 (Smad4)	MUC1	MUC2	β-Catenin	MMP-7	MTI-MMP
NNE	−	+	−	++++	UNK	+	++++	−	−
BilIN-1	−	+	−	++++	++	+	++++	+	−
BilIN-2	+	+++	+	+++	++	+	+++	++	++
BilIN-3	+	++	+	++	++	+	++	++	+++
BilIN-CC	++	+++	++++	+	++++	+	+	++++	++++
IPNB-1	+	++	++	+++	UNK	++	+++	+	UNK
IPNB-2	+++	+++	+++	++	−	+++	++	+	−
IPNB-CC	++++	++++	+++	+		++	++++	+	+

Abbreviations: BilIN-1, low-grade dysplasia; BilIN-2, high-grade dysplasia; BilIN-3, carcinoma in situ; BilIN-CC, cholangiocarcinoma with BilIN features; IPNB-1, dysplasia; IPNB-2, carcinoma in situ; IPNB-CC, cholangiocarcinoma with IPNB features. NNE, non-neoplastic epithelium; UNK, unknown; −, no expression; +, focal expression; ++, minimal expression; +++, moderate expression; ++++, extensive expression.

invasive and metastatic potential of these lesions and their worse prognosis. Additionally, lesions of the BilIN lineage express the mucin core protein MUC1 rather than MUC2, perhaps favoring a more invasive phenotype.

IPNB and IPMN demonstrate gradual increases in *cyclin D1* and *p21* expression throughout the transition to malignant phenotypes. The expression of *DPC4* and adhesion molecules seems to decline in parallel. Both lesions gain *p53* mutations during the progression from dysplasia to carcinoma in situ and eventually to invasive CC. The production of mucin proteins is associated with the more favorable MUC2 intestinal variant. Lower levels of MMP-7 and MT1-MMP may contribute to the improved prognosis in IPNB. The reciprocal relationship between *E-cadherin* and β-catenin expression and MMP-7 and MT1-MMP production suggests an important relationship between tumor invasiveness and its malignant potential.[18] IPNB-related mucinous carcinomas may have a more favorable biology because they preserve *E-cadherin* and β-catenin expression. This preservation may limit overexpression of matrix metalloproteinases (MMP-7 and MT1-MMP) that promote invasion and metastases. Although the exact mechanism of transition from IPNB to either mucinous or tubular adenocarcinoma has yet to be elucidated, the differential acquisition of mutations and loss of cell-adhesion properties offers one simplistic, but possible explanation.

Understanding the critical mechanisms of cholangiocarcinogenesis has the potential to improve screening techniques in high-risk populations, lead to the development of novel targeted therapies, improve the accuracy and prognosis of staging systems, and select patients who may benefit from adjuvant therapies. Classification of CC into those arising from BilIN and IPNB may help define further the biologic behavior of these neoplasms. Given the rarity of CC, it is unlikely that these concepts ever will be validated within the context of randomized, controlled trials. Most future observations and insight into this deadly disease will be obtained from case series, banked tissue analysis, and experiments with relevant cell lines. The authors believe that subsequent studies of CC should include documentation of BilIN and IPNB premalignant lesions and related biomarkers to assess their significance further. Clarifying these pathways may provide with an opportunity to improve the dismal prognosis of this rare disease in the future.

REFERENCES

1. DeOliveira ML, Cunningham SC, Cameron JL, et al. Cholangiocarcinoma: thirty-one-year experience with 564 patients at a single institution. Ann Surg 2007; 245(5):755–62.
2. Hejna M, Pruckmayer M, Raderer M. The role of chemotherapy and radiation in the management of biliary cancer: a review of the literature. Eur J Cancer 1998; 34(7):977–86.
3. Reid BJ, Barrett MT, Galipeau PC, et al. Barrett's esophagus: ordering the events that lead to cancer. Eur J Cancer Prev 1996;5(Suppl 2):57–65.
4. Valenzuela M, Julian TB. Ductal carcinoma in situ: biology, diagnosis, and new therapies. Clin Breast Cancer 2007;7(9):676–81.
5. McArdle JE, Lewin KJ, Randall G, et al. Distribution of dysplasias and early invasive carcinoma in Barrett's esophagus. Hum Pathol 1992;23(5):479–82.
6. Vogelstein B, Fearon ER, Hamilton SR, et al. Genetic alterations during colorectal-tumor development. N Engl J Med 1988;319(9):525–32.
7. Zen Y, Adsay NV, Bardadin K, et al. Biliary intraepithelial neoplasia: an international interobserver agreement study and proposal for diagnostic criteria. Mod Pathol 2007;20(6):701–9.

8. Chen MF, Jan YY, Chen TC. Clinical studies of mucin-producing cholangiocellular carcinoma: a study of 22 histopathology-proven cases. Ann Surg 1998;227(1):63–9.

9. Shimonishi T, Zen Y, Chen TC, et al. Increasing expression of gastrointestinal phenotypes and p53 along with histologic progression of intraductal papillary neoplasia of the liver. Hum Pathol 2002;33(5):503–11.

10. Nakanishi Y, Zen Y, Kondo S, et al. Expression of cell cycle-related molecules in biliary premalignant lesions: biliary intraepithelial neoplasia and biliary intraductal papillary neoplasm. Hum Pathol 2008;39(8):1153–61.

11. Zen Y, Sasaki M, Fujii T, et al. Different expression patterns of mucin core proteins and cytokeratins during intrahepatic cholangiocarcinogenesis from biliary intrae-pithelial neoplasia and intraductal papillary neoplasm of the bile duct—an immu-nohistochemical study of 110 cases of hepatolithiasis. J Hepatol 2006;44(2): 350–8.

12. Higashi M, Yonezawa S, Ho JJ, et al. Expression of MUC1 and MUC2 mucin anti-gens in intrahepatic bile duct tumors: its relationship with a new morphological classification of cholangiocarcinoma. Hepatology 1999;30(6):1347–55.

13. Alao JP. The regulation of cyclin D1 degradation: roles in cancer development and the potential for therapeutic invention. Mol Cancer 2007;6(24):1–16.

14. Kornmann M, Ishiwata T, Itakura J, et al. Increased cyclin D1 in human pancreatic cancer is associated with decreased postoperative survival. Oncology 1998; 55(4):363–9.

15. Sugimachi K, Aishima S, Taguchi K, et al. The role of overexpression and gene amplification of cyclin D1 in intrahepatic cholangiocarcinoma. J Hepatol 2001; 35(1):74–9.

16. Shu XO, Moore DB, Cai Q, et al. Association of cyclin D1 genotype with breast cancer risk and survival. Cancer Epidemiol Biomarkers Prev 2005;14(1):91–7.

17. Kang YK, Kim WH, Jang JJ. Expression of G1-S modulators (p53, p16, p27, cy-clin D1, Rb) and Smad4/Dpc4 in intrahepatic cholangiocarcinoma. Hum Pathol 2002;33(9):877–83.

18. Itatsu K, Zen Y, Ohira S, et al. Immunohistochemical analysis of the progression of flat and papillary preneoplastic lesions in intrahepatic cholangiocarcinogenesis in hepatolithiasis. Liver Int 2007;27(9):1174–84.

19. Biankin A, Kench JG, Biankin SA, et al. Pancreatic intraepithelial neoplasia in association with intraductal papillary mucinous neoplasms of the pancreas: impli-cations for disease progression and recurrence. Am J Surg Pathol 2004;28(9): 1184–92.

20. Waga S, Hannon GJ, Beach D, et al. The p21 inhibitor of cyclin-dependent kinases controls DNA replication by interaction with PCNA. Nature 1994; 369(6481):574–8.

21. Hahn S, Schutte M, Hoque AT, et al. DPC4, a candidate tumor suppressor gene at human chromosome 18q21.1. Science 1996;271(5247):350–3.

22. Hahn S, Bartsch D, Schroers A, et al. Mutations of the DPC4/Smad4 gene in biliary tract carcinoma. Cancer Res 1998;58(6):1124–6.

23. Argani P, Shaukat A, Kaushal M, et al. Differing rates of loss of DPC4 expression and of p53 overexpression among carcinomas of the proximal and distal bile ducts. Cancer 2001;91(7):1332–41.

24. Wilentz R, Iacobuzio-Donahue CA, Argani P, et al. Loss of expression of Dpc4 in pancreatic intraepithelial neoplasia: evidence that DPC4 inactivation occurs late in neoplastic progression. Cancer Res 2000;60(7):2002–6.

25. Kang Y, Kim WH, Lee HW, et al. Mutation of p53 and K-ras, and loss of heterozy-gosity of APC in intrahepatic cholangiocarcinoma. Lab Invest 1999;79(4):477–83.

26. Teh M, Wee A, Raju GC. An immunohistochemical study of p53 protein in gallbladder and extrahepatic bile duct/ampullary carcinomas. Cancer 1994;74(5):1542–5.
27. Washington K, Gottfried MR. Expression of p53 in adenocarcinoma of the gallbladder and bile ducts. Liver 1996;16(2):99–104.
28. Horie S, Endo K, Kawasaki H, et al. Overexpression of MDM2 protein in intrahepatic cholangiocarcinoma: relationship with p53 overexpression, Ki-67 labeling, and clinicopathological features. Virchows Arch 2000;437(1):25–30.
29. Diamantis I, Karamitopoulou E, Perentes E, et al. p53 protein immunoreactivity in extrahepatic bile duct and gallbladder cancer: correlation with tumor grade and survival. Hepatology 1995;22(3):774–9.
30. Suto T, Sugai T, Nakamura S, et al. Assessment of the expression of p53, MIB-1 (Ki-67 antigen), and argyrophilic nucleolar organizer regions in carcinoma of the extrahepatic bile duct. Cancer 1998;82(1):86–95.
31. Tokumoto N, Ikeda S, Ishizaki Y, et al. Immunohistochemical and mutational analyses of Wnt signaling components and target genes in intrahepatic cholangiocarcinomas. Int J Oncol 2005;27(4):973–80.
32. Takahashi Y, Kawate S, Watanabe M, et al. Amplification of c-myc and cyclin D1 genes in primary and metastatic carcinomas of the liver. Pathol Int 2007;57(7):437–42.
33. Yonezawa S, Sato E. Expression of mucin antigens in human cancers and its relationship with malignancy potential. Pathol Int 1997;47(12):813–30.
34. Regimbald L, Pilarski LM, Longenecker BM, et al. The breast mucin MUC1 as a novel adhesion ligand for endothelial intercellular adhesion molecule 1 in breast cancer. Cancer Res 1996;56(18):4244–9.
35. Makiguchi Y, Hinoda Y, Imai K. Effect of MUC1 mucin, an anti-adhesion molecule, on tumor cell growth. Jpn J Cancer Res 1996;87(5):505–11.
36. Wesseling J, van der Valk SW, Vos HL, et al. Episialin (MUC1) overexpression inhibits integrin-mediated cell adhesion to extracellular matrix components. J Cell Biol 1995;129(1):255–65.
37. Kondo K, Kohno N, Yokoyama A, et al. Decreased MUC1 expression induces E-cadherin-mediated cell adhesion of breast cancer cell lines. Cancer Res 1998;58(9):2014–9.
38. Sasaki M, Nakanuma Y, Kim YS. Characterization of apomucin expression in intrahepatic cholangiocarcinomas and their precursor lesions: an immunohistochemical study. Hepatology 1996;24(5):1074–8.
39. Adsay NV, Merati K, Andea A, et al. The dichotomy in the preinvasive neoplasia to invasive carcinoma sequence in the pancreas: differential expression of MUC1 and MUC2 supports the existence of two separate pathways of carcinogenesis. Mod Pathol 2002;15(10):1087–95.
40. Shibahara H, Tamada S, Goto M, et al. Pathologic features of mucin-producing bile duct tumors: two histopathologic categories as counterparts of pancreatic intraductal papillary-mucinous neoplasms. Am J Surg Pathol 2004;28(3):327–38.
41. Pecina-Slaus N. Tumor suppressor gene E-cadherin and its role in normal and malignant cells. Cancer Cell Int 2003;3(1):1–7.
42. Crawford HC, Fingleton BM, Rudolph-Owen LA, et al. The metalloproteinase matrilysin is a target of beta-catenin transactivation in intestinal tumors. Oncogene 1999;18(18):2883–91.
43. He TC, Sparks AB, Rago C, et al. Identification of c-MYC as a target of the APC pathway. Science 1998;281(5382):1509–12.
44. Tetsu O, McCormick F. Beta-catenin regulates expression of cyclin D1 in colon carcinoma cells. Nature 1999;398(6726):422–6.

45. Hirohashi S. Inactivation of the E-cadherin-mediated cell adhesion system in human cancers. Am J Pathol 1998;153(2):333–9.

46. Sugimachi K, Taguchi K, Aishima S, et al. Altered expression of beta-catenin without genetic mutation in intrahepatic cholangiocarcinoma. Mod Pathol 2001; 14(9):900–5.

47. Itatsu K, Zen Y, Yamaguchi J, et al. Expression of matrix metalloproteinase 7 is an unfavorable postoperative prognostic factor in cholangiocarcinoma of the perihilar, hilar, and extrahepatic bile ducts. Hum Pathol 2008;39(5):710–9.

48. Miwa S, Miyagawa S, Soeda J, et al. Matrix metalloproteinase-7 expression and biologic aggressiveness of cholangiocellular carcinoma. Cancer 2002;94(2): 428–34.

49. Golubkov VS, Boyd S, Savinov AY, et al. Membrane type-1 matrix metalloproteinase (MT1-MMP) exhibits an important intracellular cleavage function and causes chromosome instability. J Biol Chem 2005;280(26):25079–86.

50. Golubkov VS, Chekanov AV, Doxsey SJ, et al. Centrosomal pericentrin is a direct cleavage target of membrane type-1 matrix metalloproteinase in humans but not in mice: potential implications for tumorigenesis. J Biol Chem 2005;280(51): 42237–41.

Multimodality Imaging of Biliary Malignancies

Mandip S. Gakhal, MD*, Vinay K. Gheyi, MD, Rachel E. Brock, MD,
Glenn S. Andrews, MD

KEYWORDS

- Biliary malignancies • Biliary cancer
- Cholangiocarcinoma • Radiology • Imaging

Detection, accurate staging, and optimal management of biliary malignancies continue to present a significant challenge. Cholangiocarcinoma is relatively rare, but has a very poor prognosis. Surgery is the only curative treatment, and survival times are improving with more aggressive surgical treatment. This article reviews the current capabilities and roles of the various imaging modalities available in clinical practice, and discusses their integrated use at initial presentation, particularly with respect to potential surgical management of central hilar and intrahepatic cholangiocarcinoma. The main imaging modalities include MRI, CT, ultrasound, positron emission tomography (PET), and conventional cholangiography. Alternative and emerging imaging methods, problematic diagnostic imaging issues, and other rarer bile duct malignancies are also briefly discussed.

IMAGING GOALS

The goal of initial imaging with respect to surgical oncology evaluation of cholangiocarcinoma and other biliary malignancies is to accurately identify and then stage the extent of disease. Specifically, the critical aspect is identifying all patients in whom complete surgical resection is possible. The key parameters adapted from the staging criteria are listed in a simplified checklist format in **Table 1**.[1–3]

Imaging findings that typically render a tumor surgically unresectable include involvement of bilateral hepatic ducts and secondary biliary radicles, atrophy of one lobe with involvement of contralateral portal vein, atrophy of one lobe and contralateral secondary biliary radicle or portal vein involvement, proper hepatic artery invasion, encasement or occlusion of main portal vein before its bifurcation, portal vein involvement of one lobe and hepatic artery involvement of the other lobe, bilateral involvement of the lobar hepatic arteries, vascular invasion of one lobe and bile duct involvement of the other lobe, extensive regional adenopathy, and distant metastases.[2]

Department of Radiology, Christiana Care Health System, 4755 Ogletown Stanton Road, Newark, DE 19718, USA
* Corresponding author.
E-mail address: mgakhal@christianacare.org (M.S. Gakhal).

Surg Oncol Clin N Am 18 (2009) 225–239
doi:10.1016/j.soc.2008.12.009
1055-3207/08/$ – see front matter © 2009 Elsevier Inc. All rights reserved.

surgonc.theclinics.com

Table 1
Checklist of structures and key parameters in hilar and intrahepatic cholangiocarcinoma that should be evaluated and reported on imaging studies, thereby allowing the surgeon to determine resectability

Mass	Size, location
Bile ducts	Longitudinal and radial extent
	Degree of involvement of second-order biliary radicles
	Duct anatomy and variants
Vascular	Portal vein; main versus lobar branches
	Hepatic veins, inferior vena cava
	Proper hepatic artery, lobar hepatic artery, other
	Vessel anatomy and variants
Liver	Lobar atrophy/hypertrophy
	Direct parenchyma invasion
Nodes	Local, regional, distant
Metastases	Liver, distant

MRI AND MAGNETIC RESONANCE CHOLANGIOGRAPHY

MRI and magnetic resonance cholangiography (MRC) currently represent the most comprehensive imaging examinations for evaluating cholangiocarcinoma, and should be performed before any biliary drainage procedure if feasible.[2] Routine MRC protocols include fast T2 and heavily T2-weighted fluid-sensitive sequences that are acquired in the range of a 3- to 20-second breathhold depending on the parameters. High-resolution non-breathhold three-dimensional heavily T2-weighted sequences with respiratory triggering can be obtained within a few minutes and are also becoming standard, from which maximum intensity projection cholangiographic images can be generated and rotationally viewed at any user-selected angle or axis (Video 1); access video in online version of article at http://www.surgonc.theclinics.com. The MRI sequences include breathhold T1-weighted in and out of phase gradient echo, and fast spin echo T2-weighted images. Dynamic breathhold multiphase preintravenous and postintravenous gadolinium images in the arterial, venous, interstitial, and delayed phases are obtained using a fast three-dimensional gradient echo T1-weighted sequence. The use of all the aforementioned sequences in combination with technical developments, such as parallel imaging, multichannel coil arrays, and high field magnets, has led to steady improvements in speed and resolution. Despite the availability of such techniques as navigator triggering and other compensatory measures, a cooperative patient with ability to hold their breath is still necessary and key to generating high-quality diagnostic images, and when not achievable should lead to selection of CT as the primary or supplemental examination. CT is also indicated in patients with absolute contraindication to MRI, such as cardiac pacing device, intraocular metallic foreign body, and some intracranial aneurysm clips.

MRI can reliably identify the site of biliary ductal narrowing and evaluate for lithiasis, ductal neoplasm, liver invasion and metastases, local nodal spread, and extent of vascular involvement. The MRI appearance of the bile duct malignancy is related to its morphologic subtypes, which include mass-forming, periductal infiltrating, intraductal, and mixed.[3,4] In general, on the unenhanced images the malignancy appears as hypointense to isointense on T1-weighted images relative to liver parenchyma, and has more variable signal on T2-weighted images ranging from mildly hyperintense to hypointense. On the postcontrast images the mass-forming malignancies typically demonstrate initial peripheral enhancement, with more diffuse enhancement on delayed images. Although there is overlap with other tumors, such as colorectal metastases, hypointense T2 signal reflecting fibrosis with corresponding delayed enhancement is relatively characteristic of cholangiocarcinoma, along with more frequent peripheral bile duct dilation, and when these features are present they can aid in refining the differential diagnosis (**Fig. 1**).[5] The periductal infiltrating malignancies, when small and localized, manifest as focal wall thickening, which avidly enhances (**Fig. 2**). Larger central and hilar masses are more variable in their imaging features on both unenhanced and postcontrast sequences. They can be difficult to demarcate given their elongated, branchlike pattern of growth and confluence with adjacent structures.

In a study by Hanninen and colleagues,[6] MRI-MRC accuracy for assessment of tumor status, periductal infiltration, and lymph node metastases was 90%, 87%, and 66%, respectively, similar to other studies. MRI has been demonstrated to be more effective than endoscopic retrograde cholangiography (ERC) in delineating extent of hilar cholangiocarcinoma.[7] Level of obstruction and extent of bile duct involvement has been predicted by MRI with accuracies from 88% to 96%.[3] Dynamic

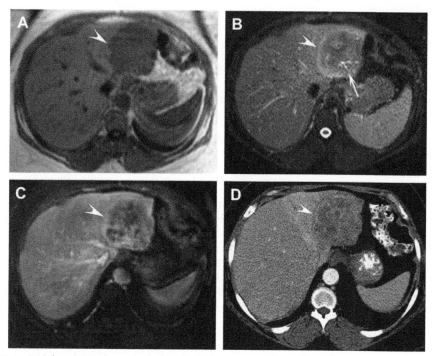

Fig. 1. Peripheral intrahepatic cholangiocarcinoma on MRI and CT. (*A*) Axial T1-weighted image demonstrates the cholangiocarcinoma (*arrowhead*) to be hypointense relative to liver parenchyma. (*B*) On axial T2-weighted images the mass (*arrowhead*) is mildly hyperintense to hypointense compared with normal liver parenchyma. A few dilated peripheral biliary radicles are also demonstrated (*arrow*). (*C* and *D*) Contrast-enhanced MRI and CT images, respectively, demonstrate heterogeneous enhancement in the cholangiocarcinoma (*arrowhead*).

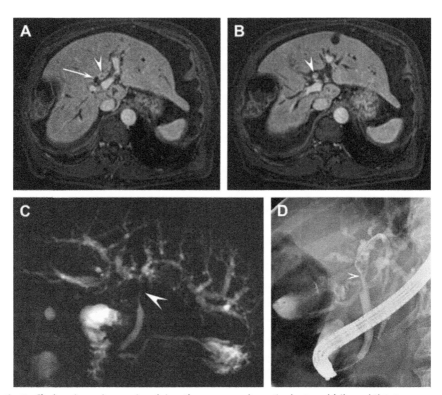

Fig. 2. Cholangiocarcinoma involving the common hepatic duct and hilum. (*A*) Intravenous gadolinium-enhanced gradient echo T1-weighted image demonstrates the tumor as avidly enhancing circumferential mural thickening of the left hepatic duct (*arrowhead*). Normal-appearing right hepatic duct at this level (*arrow*). (*B*) Tumor at the common hepatic duct level manifests as focal mural and intraluminal enhancement with severe lumen narrowing (*arrowhead*). MRC (*C*) and endoscopic retrograde cholangiography (*D*) images demonstrate bile duct narrowing corresponding to the sites of abnormal enhancement (*arrowhead*).

contrast-enhanced MRI is comparable with angiography in assessment of portal vein and arterial invasion. MRI can help guide the choice of ERC versus percutaneous transhepatic cholangiography (PTC), and also facilitate their success. In those receiving percutaneous interventions, MRI has been shown correctly to predict extent of biliary involvement in 96%, and the therapeutic plan anticipated with MRI matched the one actually used in 83%.[8] MRI also has use in evaluation of postoperative complications, such as biliary-enteric anastomotic strictures, biliary lithiasis, and neoplasm recurrence.

CT SCANNING

Current multidetector CT technology allows for rapid high-resolution multiphase scanning of large anatomic regions without motion artifacts. Power injectors in conjunction with contrast bolus detection and triggering mechanisms deliver precisely controlled rate and amount of iodinated intravenous contrast, optimizing protocol standardization and reproducibility. Although protocols and equipment vary between institutions, general recommendations for presurgical CT evaluation of cholangiocarcinoma include contrast-enhanced imaging using thin collimation in the arterial, portal venous, and equilibrium or delayed phases.

The acquired source data are typically reconstructed between 1- and 5-mm slice thickness for transverse images depending on its intended use, with coronal and sagittal reformations as necessary. The thin-section volumetric transverse images are also routinely reviewed in an interactive multiplanar mode. The effects of reformatted images on diagnosis, staging, and treatment planning have been studied. Park and colleagues[9] found that addition of coronal images to standard transverse images in extrahepatic bile duct carcinoma resulted in no significant increase in the accuracy of preoperative tumor staging, but had added value in optimally displaying the imaging findings and delineating anatomic relationships for surgical planning. Kakihara and colleagues[10] found improvement in image interpretation confidence levels and efficacy for local tumor extension of biliary carcinoma using curved planar reformations along the long axis of bile ducts and short axis multiplanar reformations perpendicular to the ducts.

The CT characteristics of cholangiocarcinoma are variable depending on location, size, tumor morphology, and timing of image acquisition. Similar to MRI, mass-forming peripheral cholangiocarcinoma can have peripheral rim enhancement on arterial and venous phase CT, with further enhancement on the delayed images. Asayama and colleagues[11] found that delayed enhancement on CT in greater than two thirds of a tumor was an independent adverse prognostic indicator with lower patient survival rate. Intrahepatic intraductal tumors result in dilation of the ducts, the contents of which may be higher in attenuation than simple fluid. Hilar and infiltrating periductal cholangiocarcinoma both appear as ill-defined or focal masses and are initially hypovascular with more heterogeneous enhancement on the delayed images compared with the peripheral tumors. Liver atrophy, capsular retraction, bile duct irregularity, and lumen obliteration are useful signs.[12] CT evaluation of central biliary carcinoma requires detection of subtle changes in anatomic planes, attenuation, and enhancement compared with normal bile duct walls, bile, periportal fat, and liver parenchyma (**Fig. 3**). Lumen caliber, mural thickness and margins, morphology, patency and extent of perimeter tumor contact must be assessed for the vascular structures, similar to the method of analysis with MRI (**Fig. 4**).

Accuracy for detection of cholangiocarcinoma with modern CT technology is between 86% and 100%.[8] Preoperative evaluation of hilar cholangiocarcinoma by Unno and colleagues[13] using 16-channel CT and multiphase contrast-enhanced images, where tumor mostly manifested as a hypervascular lesion in the late arterial phase, yielded 80.9% accuracy for diagnosis of spread along the axis of the bile duct, and 100% accuracy for diagnosis of tumor extension into neighboring tissues, such as the hepatic parenchyma and vascular structures. They acknowledged lesser success caused by artifacts in patients with indwelling biliary drainage tubes, where accuracy was reduced to 62.5% (**Fig. 5**). In that particular study, although the sensitivity for lymph nodes metastases was 100%, the specificity was only 35.7%, with false-negative in 64.3%, and a negative predictive value of 52.6%. Endo and colleagues[14] studied use of three-dimensional imaging with multidetector CT and advanced post-processing software in operative planning for hilar cholangiocarcinoma. In addition to the usual iodinated intravenous contrast injection they also acquired contrast-enhanced images of the bile ducts, either through direct injection of percutaneous biliary catheters, or in those with internal stents or no catheters by administering an intravenous agent that has detectable biliary excretion. They achieved 85% to 87% accuracy for longitudinal tumor extension; 100% sensitivity, 80% specificity, and 87% accuracy for portal vein invasion; and 75% sensitivity, 91% specificity, and

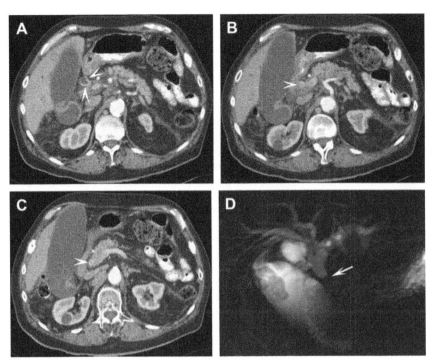

Fig. 3. Cholangiocarcinoma in the inferior common hepatic duct and a portion of the common bile duct. (*A*) Contrast-enhanced axial CT image shows malignancy near its upper margin manifesting as eccentric mural thickening and enhancement (*arrowheads*) of the inferior common hepatic duct. (*B*) Most of the cholangiocarcinoma appears as solid duct enhancement and expansion with obliteration of the duct lumen (*arrowhead*). (*C*) Near its inferior margin the cholangiocarcinoma appears at circumferential wall thickening and severe narrowing of the lumen (*arrowhead*). (*D*) T2-weighted thick slab coronal image demonstrates the MRC appearance of the same tumor with narrowing of the inferior common hepatic duct and common bile duct (*arrow*).

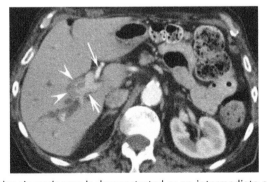

Fig. 4. Central cholangiocarcinoma is demonstrated as an intermediate-attenuation region (*arrowheads*) surrounding a central high-attenuation dot that represents an encased and narrowed right hepatic artery branch. The mass contacts the portal vein (*short arrow*) near its bifurcation with greater involvement of the right portal vein branch compared with the left, along with greater bile duct dilation in the right lobe. Normal left hepatic artery (*long arrow*) is distant from the mass.

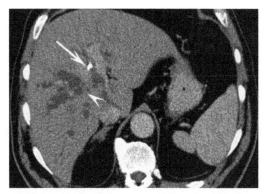

Fig. 5. CT imaging following endoscopic stent placement for biliary obstruction caused by central cholangiocarcinoma, with the upper portion of the stent extending into the left lobe ducts (*arrow*). In this case there was imaging evidence of malignancy peripheral to second-order bile ducts in the right lobe (*arrowhead*). It was difficult, however, to evaluate reliably the tumor extent in the decompressed left-sided bile ducts. The tumor proved to be unresectable on surgical exploration of the left bile ducts.

87% accuracy for hepatic arterial invasion. In another prior study by Cha and colleagues,[15] CT was shown to have an accuracy of 86% and 93% in predicting portal venous and hepatic arterial invasion, respectively. Aloia and colleagues[16] showed that high-resolution CT could predict resectability of hilar cholangiocarcinoma with a sensitivity of 94% and specificity of 79%. The negative predictive value was 92% and positive predictive value was 85%. In their study the cases where CT incorrectly predicted resectability consisted of subcentimeter peritoneal disease, subcentimeter liver metastasis, and small bile duct involvement.

CONVENTIONAL CHOLANGIOGRAPHY

ERC and PTC are invasive procedures but provide higher-resolution images of the bile ducts, compared with MRC and CT. The ability to distend ducts and increase their visibility by direct intraluminal contrast injection is a valuable advantage over cross-sectional imaging methods. Conventional cholangiography only provides a composite image of the biliary lumen, however, with overlap of ducts and no information about surrounding structures. It can be difficult on ERC and PTC adequately to opacify bile ducts peripheral to the site of obstruction, and intraductal debris may simulate neoplasm. If feasible, ERC is typically chosen over PTC as the initial option. PTC is performed for failed ERC, complex biliary obstruction, or drainage of biliary ductal territories not amenable to endoscopic approach. Complications of ERC and PTC are uncommon but range from cholangitis, sepsis, pancreatitis, and hemorrhage to death. The risks must be weighed, however, against the benefits of relieving biliary obstruction and the opportunity to establish a diagnosis.

ULTRASOUND

Ultrasonography is widely accepted as initial screening imaging modality in patients presenting with obstructive jaundice. The sensitivity of detecting dilatation of the bile ducts by ultrasonography is excellent. The important sonographic diagnostic hallmark is the detection of dilated bile ducts followed to the point of caliber change, which indicates the point of obstruction. Significant advances in resolving power of sonography equipment has enabled visualization of normal nondilated bile ducts on the current scanners. In the past, only the dilated bile ducts were visualized and were therefore considered to be abnormal. It is crucial to avoid interpreting the normal bile ducts as dilated just because they can be visualized. The intrahepatic ducts are considered to be normal if the cross-sectional diameter of the intrahepatic ducts is 2 mm or less and does not exceed 40% of diameter of the accompanying portal vein.[17]

The two well-documented strengths of ultrasonography in cholangiocarcinoma evaluation are its ability to determine reliably the level of biliary obstruction and the determination of vascular invasion. Various studies have documented accurate assessment of level of biliary obstruction by ultrasonography.[18,19] A total of 93% sensitivity and 99% specificity with a positive predictive value of 97% for portal vein involvement was demonstrated in a series of 63 consecutive patients with hilar cholangiocarcinoma.[20] In a series of 22 patients with hilar cholangiocarcinoma subjected to surgery, duplex ultrasonography correctly demonstrated portal vein patency in 86% of patients. By comparison, arteriography was accurate in 82% of cases.[18] Both ultrasound and MRI provide comparable results for diagnosis of hepatic vein involvement by tumor at the level of hepatic venous confluence in potential candidates for hepatic resection. MRI and CT are superior to ultrasound for lesion detection and characterization, however, although ultrasound is cheaper and more readily available.

Ultrasonography for overall assessment of cholangiocarcinoma remains deficient compared with CT and MRI. Ultrasonography is operator dependent and the results vary according to the degree of operator expertise and institutional experience. Studies have documented limitations of ultrasonography in estimation of tumor spread and determination of resectability.[17] Likewise, suboptimal sensitivity of ultrasound in detection of tumor infiltration of the hepatic artery (43%), peritoneal deposits (33%), metastases to regional lymph nodes (37%), and detection of satellite liver lesions (66%) has been described.[19]

Two morphologically different ultrasound appearances have been described with intrahepatic cholangiocarcinomas. There is a nodular form that presents as a solitary intrahepatic mass and an infiltrative form that is more difficult to evaluate and presents with diffusely abnormal liver echotexture. The nodular form consists of a hepatic mass of variable echogenicity, although tumors less than 3 cm tend to be hypoechoic and tumors greater than 3 cm are more hyperechoic.[17] This increase in echogenicity of the tumor has been well documented in literature.[21] Sonographically, hepatocellular carcinoma and metastasis may have appearance similar to intrahepatic cholangiocarcinoma. Presence of biliary ductal dilatation peripheral to the intrahepatic mass is more commonly seen with intrahepatic cholangiocarcinoma and is rarely seen with hepatocellular carcinoma.[21,22] Hepatic metastases are more difficult to distinguish from cholangiocarcinoma, and both tumors can present as biliary intraluminal masses.

The most frequent finding of hilar cholangiocarcinomas is intrahepatic biliary duct dilatation, and a ductal mass may not be apparent on the ultrasound examination. The association of segmental dilatation and nonunion of the right and left hepatic ducts at the hepatic hilum are suggestive of Klatskin's tumor.[17] Dilatation of intrahepatic bile ducts associated with normal-caliber extrahepatic ducts also suggests Klatskin's tumor, but it is necessary to exclude lymphadenopathy or other causes of extrinsic obstruction of the bile ducts at the hepatic hilum. Although in some cases a discrete mass may be present, cholangiocarcinoma more commonly presents with isoechoic infiltration of periductal tissues, and because the echotexture of infiltrating mass may resemble that of hepatic parenchyma, it may be difficult to delineate the tumor margins. Identification of such lesions depends on detecting subtle mass effect over the ductal structures and adjacent vessels. In some cases, prominent focal irregularity of the ducts related to tumor tissue may be visible.

Ultrasound evaluation is helpful for assessment of vascular involvement by the tumor. The sensitivity of ultrasound for detection of portal vein and hepatic vein involvement by the tumor is similar to MRI scan, but evaluation of hepatic artery remains technically difficult and suboptimal. Vascular assessment should use gray-scale imaging, color Doppler, and spectral Doppler ultrasound for optimum assessment of vessels. Because of the better spatial resolution of gray-scale ultrasound, morphologic findings, such as invasion, encasement, and obliteration of vascular lumen, are better depicted, whereas intratumoral vascularity may only be visualized on color Doppler imaging. Because approximation of the mass to a vessel does not necessarily mean vascular invasion, caliber alteration of the vessel and focal velocity change on spectral Doppler analysis are more specific findings.

POSITRON EMISSION TOMOGRAPHY AND POSITRON EMISSION TOMOGRAPHY–CT

There are limited studies in the literature defining the role of PET and PET-CT in the diagnosis, staging work-up, and posttreatment follow-up evaluation of cholangiocarcinoma. Further studies in larger cohorts of patients are needed to establish the exact role of this modality in imaging and management of cholangiocarcinoma.

Analysis of current literature, however, indicates that most biliary cancers are fluoro-deoxyglucose (FDG) avid.[23] The largest series evaluating the clinical use of PET in biliary cancers included 36 patients with cholangiocarcinoma and 14 patients with gallbladder carcinoma, demonstrating overall sensitivity of PET in detection of cholangiocarcinoma to be 61%.[24] The study further indicated that sensitivity of PET for detection of the nodular-type cholangiocarcinoma was 85%, and only 18% for the infiltrating morphology. Similarly, better sensitivity of detection of the intrahepatic type (95%) than the extrahepatic type (69%) was also noted by Corvera and colleagues.[23] Likewise, Jadvar and colleagues[25] also noted false-negative results for detection of infiltrating type of cholangiocarcinoma. It has been suggested that larger size of intrahepatic cholangiocarcinoma at the time of presentation may account for the better sensitivity of detection by FDG-PET.[23] Furthermore, the FDG uptake in the infiltrating types of cholangiocarcinoma is similar or only slightly increased when compared with hepatic parenchyma and the detection is further confounded by the physiologic heterogeneity of background hepatic uptake activity, thereby rendering detection of these lesions difficult or impossible.[25] The available data suggest that although the sensitivity for detection of nodular variety of cholangiocarcinoma approaches 85% to 95%, a significant number of infiltrating cholangiocarcinomas are missed by PET.[23-25] FDG uptake is not specific to malignancies, however, and false-positive results have also been described secondary to postoperative changes, acute cholangitis, and inflammatory changes from biliary stent placement.[24]

With regards to staging of cholangiocarcinoma, studies have shown that PET and PET-CT may avoid unnecessary surgery by identifying occult metastatic disease.[23-25] PET evaluation, however, lacks sufficient spatial resolution and anatomic information for assessment of local and regional extent and resection feasibility. The local extent is better evaluated with CT or MRI. PET scan may detect distant metastases, however, thereby avoiding unnecessary surgery. The series by Corvera and colleagues[23] demonstrated that PET imaging changed treatment plan in nearly one quarter patients with cholangiocarcinoma by detecting occult metastatic disease.

The studies on use of FDG PET and PET-CT in assessment of posttreatment recurrence and follow-up surveillance are limited, but preliminary data suggest that FDG

PET may be helpful in this setting. Worsening disease following treatment may be demonstrated by development of new local or distant metastatic lesions, and by increase in uptake values of previously documented lesions, specifically when CT scan or MRI scan may not show significant interval change. Similarly, PET may help to exclude recurrence at the surgical margins by demonstrating absent FDG activity, whereas CT and MRI may show ambiguous postsurgical contrast enhancement.[25] The tumors that are FDG negative, however, may be better evaluated with contrast-enhanced CT or MRI. Overall, PET and PET-CT play a complimentary role to anatomic imaging with CT or MRI, and the combined information provides the most useful data for accurate staging.

INTEGRATED MULTIMODALITY IMAGING OF BILIARY MALIGNANCY

One of the most common imaging algorithms is initial imaging work-up by a screening ultrasound or routine single-phase contrast-enhanced CT depending on the clinical presentation, which then leads either to MRI-MRC or a multiphase high-resolution CT examination, followed by selective use of PET, ERC, and PTC. CT and MRI-MRC are often complementary examinations, and if either does not fully provide the necessary diagnostic staging information, the second of the two can be performed for correlation and specific problem solving (**Fig. 6**). The addition of PET and PET-CT may alter the treatment plan by detecting unsuspected distant metastases, thereby avoiding unnecessary surgery.[23]

The perception of limitations of CT as an effective modality compared with MRI for the evaluation of cholangiocarcinoma is at least partly the result of experience with older technology and suboptimal protocols. A more recent study found no statistically significant difference in accuracy between multidetector CT and MRC for evaluating extent of biliary ductal involvement in hilar cholangiocarcinoma.[26] MRI has better contrast and tissue differentiation characteristics by use of multiple sequences, but CT has better resolution and allows multiplanar review of source data. The newer multichannel or multidetector CT scanners can generate isotropic or near isotropic voxels, which in combination with the appropriate postprocessing tools can provide information similar to MRI-MRC. Surgeons can better relate to reformatted coronal, multiplanar, or three-dimensional workstation generated images, compared with the

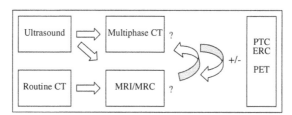

Fig. 6. Typical multimodality imaging algorithm for biliary malignancies is illustrated. Initial imaging work-up is commonly done with screening ultrasound or routine single-phase contrast-enhanced CT depending on the clinical presentation, which then leads either to MRI-MRC or a multiphase high-resolution CT examination, followed by selective use of PET, ERC, and PTC. CT and MRI-MRC are often complementary examinations, and if either does not fully provide the necessary diagnostic staging information, the second of the two can be performed for correlation and specific problem solving. CT, computed tomography; ERC, endoscopic retrograde cholangiography; MRC, magnetic resonance cholangiography; MRI, magnetic resonance imaging; PET, positron emission tomography; PTC, percutaneous transhepatic cholangiography.

traditional axial images. CT is still more widely available, and is overall a much more time efficient endeavor. Allergy to iodinated contrast and abnormal renal function can be limiting factors for CT. The prior presumed advantage of MRI with regard to patients with renal dysfunction is no longer valid, given the risk of developing nephrogenic systemic fibrosis with intravenous gadolinium administration in those with low glomerular filtration rate.

Rather than using a single imaging study multiple modalities are often used in concert. CT or MRI can be used to perform liver volume calculations, to determine feasibility of surgical resection, or precisely to document adequacy of hypertrophy and increase in volume after portal vein embolization procedure (**Fig. 7**, Video 2) (access video in online version of article at http://www.surgonc.theclinics.com). Cholangiocarcinoma occurs in 6% to 20% of patients with primary sclerosing cholangitis, and also often requires imaging with multiple modalities, because manifestations can be subtle, and detection further confounded by the underlying primary sclerosing cholangitis–induced ductal abnormalities. The imaging findings suggestive of malignancy in primary sclerosing cholangitis on all modalities include dilated ducts proximal to a stricture, polypoid ductal lesions, high-grade ductal narrowing, rapid stricture evolution, and progressive stricture with progressive ductal dilation. Beyond the cholangiocarcinoma itself, multimodality imaging can also directly demonstrate manifestations of the risk factors and associated entities, such as biliary lithiasis, clonorchiasis, recurrent pyogenic cholangitis, primary sclerosing cholangitis, and choledochal cyst. A more comprehensive armamentarium of imaging studies can be necessary in peripheral cholangiocarcinoma, because the initial biopsy typically yields adenocarcinoma, triggering the search for a primary elsewhere, which if negative, implies biliary origin. Studies include CT of chest, abdomen, and pelvis; pelvic ultrasound; and mammogram.[27] MRI and PET are also being used in this scenario with increasing frequency.

Posttreatment follow-up may also require multimodality imaging. In particular, the anatomic imaging with CT and MRI provides significant information with regards to tumor size, morphology, locoregional spread, and status of adjacent vessels. In some cases, however, it may not be possible to differentiate postsurgical changes from tumor recurrence, and PET/PET-CT may be of use if the original tumor had avid FDG uptake.

DIAGNOSTIC IMAGING CHALLENGES

Despite technologic advances and improvements, some of the long-standing imaging dilemmas still persist. It is not possible to differentiate reliably between benign and malignant biliary strictures.[2,3] Early imaging detection of cholangiocarcinoma in primary sclerosing cholangitis is problematic. Hepatobiliary fibrosis and sclerosis often cannot be distinguished from tumor. Identification of exact margins of spread of the infiltrating ductal type of cholangiocarcinoma is not always possible and typically underestimated on imaging examinations. In one recent study, evaluation of the longitudinal pattern of growth of hilar cholangiocarcinoma along the axis of the duct with CT had an accuracy ranging from 54% to 64%.[28] Superficial and microscopic extension along small bile ducts, and perineural invasion, which occurs in as much as 81% of cholangiocarcinomas,[29] is occult on current imaging studies. Early peritoneal spread can be missed on imaging, and detected only at time of surgical exploration. Hepatolithiasis is not only a risk factor for cholangiocarcinoma, but can confound its diagnosis. Both cholangiocarcinoma- and hepatolithiasis-associated cholangitis may present with biliary strictures, fibrosis, and upstream ductal dilation.[30] Cross-sectional imaging studies remain suboptimal in their ability to identify

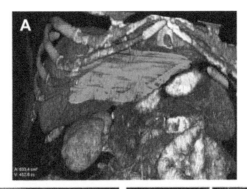

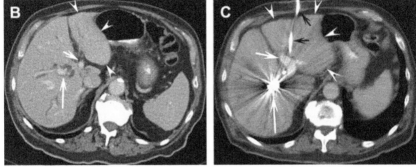

Fig. 7. (*A*) Coronal volume-rendered image demonstrates shaded surface display over the left hepatic lobe (*blue*) generated from manually drawn contours around the left hepatic lobe margins on the source images to calculate the volume for presurgical planning purposes. (*B*) CT image before right portal vein embolization demonstrates patent right portal vein branch (*long arrow*); patent left portal vein branch (*short arrow*); and baseline size of left hepatic lobe lateral segment (*arrowheads*). (*C*) CT image of the same patient 34 days following embolization procedure reveals multiple coils (*long arrow*) in the now occluded right portal vein branch; preserved patency of the left portal vein branch (*short arrow*); significant visible hypertrophy of the left hepatic lobe lateral segment (*arrowheads*); and quantitative volume increase as determined on CT from 260 to 325 mL. There has also been interval placement of an internal-external biliary drainage catheter with decompression of the previously dilated bile ducts (*black arrows*).

nodal metastases. A recent study again found CT unreliable for predicting regional nodal metastases in biliary carcinoma. Regional nodes with short axis exceeding 16 mm had a positive predictive value of 56% for the presence of metastases, whereas heterogeneous nodal enhancement had a positive predictive value of 64%.[31] In a CT study,[13] sensitivity for detecting malignant nodes was only 35.7%. PET and PET-CT may prove more sensitive in detecting pathologic nodes.

Recognizing the limitations of imaging studies is equally as important as understanding their use. It cannot be overemphasized that no patient should be denied the chance for surgical resection based on uncertain or equivocal imaging findings. If there is any doubt about resectability, the patient should proceed onto at least exploratory surgical evaluation.

ALTERNATIVE, INVESTIGATIONAL, AND EMERGING IMAGING TECHNIQUES

Numerous alternative imaging methods have been investigated, whereas others continue be researched, and a handful of them are briefly discussed herein. In patients with prior biliary drainage, three-dimensional multidetector CT cholangiography performed by direct injection of the biliary catheter has demonstrated encouraging results, with a feasibility study showing positive predictive value of 90% and negative predictive value of 100% for evaluation of biliary ductal involvement in hilar cholangiocarcinoma.[28] There is renewed interest in CT contrast agents that are directly excreted into the biliary system. Oncologic uses of dual-energy imaging with the recently developed dual-source CT scanner are being evaluated.

Administration of intravenous morphine before MRCP has been shown to increase extent of biliary distention by inducing contraction of the sphincter of Oddi, increasing duct visibility with some success,[32] and may allow for detection of more subtle abnormalities and details regarding configuration of ductal anatomy. Superparamagnetic iron oxide (ferumoxide)–based contrast MR imaging, where the contrast agent is taken up by Kupffer cells in normal hepatic parenchyma rendering it dark in signal, has been used to define better the margins between liver and intrahepatic cholangiocarcinoma.[33] A similar contrast agent, but with smaller size paramagnetic iron oxide particles that are taken up by only normal lymph nodes rendering them dark in signal, has potential use in identifying unenlarged but malignant nodes. Imaging with new MRI scanners at the higher magnetic field strength of 7 T, compared with the 1.5- and 3-T scanners currently under routine clinical use, will likely prove to be of benefit in the near future.

Direct cholangioscopy and intraductal endoscopic ultrasound are currently in limited use. Oncologic applications of molecular imaging are in the early experimental phases of development.

OTHER BILIARY MALIGNANCIES

Biliary cystadenocarcinoma is rare but the diagnosis can be suggested based on the imaging appearance, because it presents as a complex heterogeneous cystic mass with septations, mural thickening, nodular or solid components, and enhancing regions. Biliary intraductal papillary mucinous tumors have been discussed in the literature as a distinct entity, with the mass itself resembling the intraductal form of cholangiocarcinoma, but with pronounced biliary ductal dilation that can occur both proximal and distal to the mass because of excessive mucin production. Mixed hepatocellular and cholangiocarcinoma can also occur, and should be considered as an etiology when a hypervascular component is encountered in an otherwise typical-appearing cholangiocarcinoma, with other supportive data including abnormal alpha fetoprotein and a cirrhotic liver.[34]

SUMMARY

MRI-MRC and CT currently constitute the main studies for imaging cholangiocarcinoma, with evolving role of PET, and selective use of conventional cholangiography and screening ultrasound. Appropriate combined use of the various available imaging modalities is effective in staging the malignancy in most instances, thereby aiding the surgeon in clinical decision-making, patient management, and in particular determining the potential for curative surgical resection.

APPENDIX: SUPPLEMENTARY MATERIAL

Supplementary material can be found, in the online version, at doi:10.1016/j.soc.2008.12.009.

REFERENCES

1. Jarnagin WR, Fong Y, DeMatteo RP, et al. Staging, resectability, and outcome in 225 patients with hilar cholangiocarcinoma. Ann Surg 2001;234(4):507–17 [discussion: 517–9].
2. Slattery JM, Sahani DV. What is the current state-of-the-art imaging for detection and staging of cholangiocarcinoma? Oncologist 2006;11(8):913–22 [review].
3. Zech C, Schoenberg S, Reiser M. Cross-sectional imaging of biliary tumors: current clinical status and future developments. Eur Radiol 2004;14(7):1174–87.
4. Patel T. Cholangiocarcinoma. Nat Clin Pract Gastroenterol Hepatol 2006;3(1): 33–42 [review].
5. Maetani Y, Itoh K, Watanabe C, et al. MR imaging of intrahepatic cholangiocarcinoma with pathologic correlation. AJR Am J Roentgenol 2001;176(6): 1499–507.
6. Hänninen EL, Pech M, Jonas S, et al. Magnetic resonance imaging including magnetic resonance cholangiopancreatography for tumor localization and therapy planning in malignant hilar obstructions. Acta Radiol 2005;46(5): 462–70.
7. Yeh T-S, Jan Y-Y, Tseng J-H, et al. Malignant perihilar biliary obstruction: magnetic resonance cholangiopancreatographic findings. Am J Gastroenterol 2000;95(2): 432–40.
8. Lopera JE, Soto JA, Múnera F. Malignant hilar and perihilar biliary obstruction: use of MR cholangiography to define the extent of biliary ductal involvement and plan percutaneous interventions. Radiology 2001;220(1):90–6.
9. Park M, Lee D, Kim M, et al. Preoperative staging accuracy of multidetector row computer tomography of extrahepatic bile duct carcinoma. J Comput Assist Tomogr 2006;30(3):362–7.
10. Kakihara D, Yoshimitsu K, Irie H, et al. Usefulness of the long-axis and short-axis reformatted images of multidetector-row CT in evaluating T-factor of the surgically resected pancreatobiliary malignancies. Eur J Radiol 2007;63(1):96–104.
11. Asayama Y, Yoshimitsu K, Irie H, et al. Delayed-phase dynamic CT enhancement as a prognostic factor for mass-forming intrahepatic cholangiocarcinoma. Radiology 2006;238(1):150–5.
12. Kim J, Kim T, Eun H. CT findings of cholangiocarcinoma associated with recurrent pyogenic cholangitis. AJR Am J Roentgenol 2006;187(6):1571–7.
13. Unno M, Okumoto T, Katayose Y, et al. Preoperative assessment of hilar cholangiocarcinoma by multidetector row computed tomography. J Hepatobiliary Pancreat Surg 2007;14(5):434–40.
14. Endo I, Shimada H, Sugita M, et al. Role of three-dimensional imaging in operative planning for hilar cholangiocarcinoma. Surgery 2007;142(5):666–75.
15. Cha JH, Han JK, Kim TK, et al. Preoperative evaluation of Klatskin tumor: accuracy of spiral CT in determining vascular invasion as a sign of unresectability. Abdom Imaging 2000;25(5):500–7.
16. Aloia T, Charnsangavej C, Faria S, et al. High-resolution computed tomography accurately predicts respectability in hilar cholangiocarcinoma. Am J Surg 2007; 193:702–6.
17. Bloom CM, Langer W, Wilson S. Role of US in the detection, characterization, and staging of cholangiocarcinoma. Radiographics 1999;19(5):1199–218.
18. Looser C, Stain SC, Baer HU, et al. Staging of hilar cholangiocarcinoma by ultrasound and duplex sonography: a comparison with angiography and operative findings. Br J Radiol 1992;65(778):871–6.

19. Neumaier CE, Bertolotto M, Perrone R, et al. Staging of hilar cholangiocarcinoma with ultrasound. J Clin Ultrasound 1995;23(3):173–8.
20. Bach AM, Hann LE, Brown KT, et al. Portal vein evaluation with US: comparison to angiography combined with CT arterial portography. Radiology 1996;201(1): 149–54.
21. Wibulpolprasert B, Dhiensiri T. Peripheral cholangiocarcinoma: sonographic evaluation. J Clin Ultrasound 1992;20(5):303–14.
22. Lee NW, Wong KP, Siu KF, et al. Cholangiography in hepatocellular carcinoma with obstructive jaundice. Clin Radiol 1984;35(2):119–23.
23. Corvera CU, Blumgart LH, Akhurst, et al. 18F-flurodeoxyglucose positron emission tomography influences management decisions in patients with biliary cancer. J Am Coll Surg 2008;206(1):57–65.
24. Anderson CD, Rice MH, Pinson CW, et al. Fluorodeoxyglucose PET imaging in the evaluation of gallbladder carcinoma and cholangiocarcinoma. J Gastrointest Surg 2004;8(1):90–7.
25. Jadvar H, Henderson RW, Conti PS. [F-18]flurodeoxyglucose positron emission tomography and positron emission tomography: computed tomography in recurrent and metastatic cholangiocarcinoma. J Comput Assist Tomogr 2007;31(2): 223–8.
26. Cho E, Park M, Yu J, et al. Biliary ductal involvement of hilar cholangiocarcinoma: multidetector computed tomography versus magnetic resonance cholangiography. J Comput Assist Tomogr 2007;31(1):72–8.
27. Miller G, Schwartz LH, D'Angelica M. The use of imaging in the diagnosis and staging of hepatobiliary malignancies. Surg Oncol Clin N Am 2007;16(2): 343–68 [review].
28. Kim H, Kim A, Hong S, et al. Biliary ductal evaluation of hilar cholangiocarcinoma: three-dimensional direct multi-detector row CT cholangiographic findings versus surgical and pathological results - feasibility study. Radiology 2006;238(1):300–8.
29. Bhuiya MR, Nimura Y, Kamiya J, et al. Clinicopathologic factors influencing survival of patients with bile duct cancer: multivariate analysis. World J Surg 1993;17(5):653–7.
30. Park H, Lee J, Kim S, et al. CT differentiation of cholangiocarcinoma from periductal fibrosis in patients with hepatolithiasis. AJR Am J Roentgenol 2006; 187(2):445–53.
31. Noji T, Kondo S, Hirano S, et al. Computer tomography evaluation of regional lymph node metastases in patients with biliary cancer. Br J Surg 2008;95(1):92–6.
32. Silva AC, Friese JL, Hara AK, et al. MR cholangiopancreatography: improved ductal distention with intravenous morphine administration. Radiographics 2004;24(3):677–87.
33. Braga HJ, Imam K, Bluemke DA. MR imaging of intrahepatic cholangiocarcinoma: use of ferumoxides for lesion localization and extension. AJR Am J Roentgenol 2001;177(1):111–4.
34. Lee WJ, Lim HK, Jang KM, et al. Radiologic spectrum of cholangiocarcinoma: emphasis on unusual manifestations and differential diagnoses. Radiographics 2001;21(Spec No):S97–116.

Percutaneous Approach to the Diagnosis and Treatment of Biliary Tract Malignancies

Mark J. Garcia, MD, FSIR*, David S. Epstein, MD, Michael A. Dignazio, MD

KEYWORDS

- Biliary • Malignancies • Percutaneous • Management
- Chemoembolization • Drainage

The role of percutaneous, transhepatic management of biliary tract malignancies is to provide diagnostic and palliative care for improving patient quality of life. The most common causes of death in patients who have unresectable disease include liver failure and cholangitis secondary to the obstruction. These patients often die 6 to 12 months after diagnosis.[1,2] Measures aimed at relieving patient symptoms include surgical, percutaneous, and endoscopic decompression of the biliary system.[3] Although surgical resection offers the only significant chance for 5-year survival, few patients are operative candidates.[4] In addition, extrahepatic malignancies are cured by surgery in less than 10% of all cases.[5] Interventional radiologists continue to develop techniques in the hope of improving quality and prolongation of life. To this end, there are several nontraditional treatments that interventional radiologists may offer in their management of biliary cancers. This article focuses on percutaneous approaches to management of biliary tract malignancies during diagnosis, including cholangiography and intraductal biopsy, treatment of malignancy via transhepatic decompression, and transarterial and transhepatic therapies.

EPIDEMIOLOGY AND ANATOMY

Malignant biliary obstruction is caused by primary and secondary diseases. Primary bile duct malignancies include cholangiocarcinoma and gallbladder cancers. Secondary malignancies include pancreatic and hepatic cancers and metastatic disease to the biliary tree or adjacent structures. All of these secondary malignancies

Division of Interventional Radiology, Christiana Care Health System, 4755 Ogletown-Stanton Road, Suite 1E10, Newark, DE 19718, USA
* Corresponding author.
E-mail address: magarcia@christianacare.org (M.J. Garcia).

Surg Oncol Clin N Am 18 (2009) 241–256
doi:10.1016/j.soc.2008.12.002
1055-3207/08/$ – see front matter © 2009 Elsevier Inc. All rights reserved.

can cause biliary obstruction by direct invasion or extrinsic compression.[6] Primary cancers or cholangiocarcinomas generally are separated anatomically as intrahepatic or extrahepatic by location (arising within the liver capsule or in the extrahepatic biliary tree from the capsule margin to the ampulla of Vater). Extrahepatic malignancies can be subdivided further into perihilar (Klatskin tumor) and distal cancers. Distal cancers involve the common bile duct from the superior margin of the pancreatic head to the ampulla of Vater.[7,8] Among cholangiocarcinomas, 5% to 10% are intrahepatic and two thirds are hilar/perihilar, with 25% of cholangiocarcinomas occurring in the distal bile ducts.[9,10] Adenocarcinoma is the most common cell type, accounting for 90% to 95% of all cholangiocarcinomas.[11] It is estimated that 4600 new cases of cholangiocarcinoma will be presented in the United States in 2008.[9]

PREPROCEDURAL EVALUATION AND MANAGEMENT

Initial preprocedural evaluation of patients who have obstructive biliary disease requiring biliary intervention requires a thorough history, physical examination, and review of all imaging and laboratory work. Malignant obstruction frequently is accompanied by jaundice, malaise, weight loss, anorexia, pruritis, acholic stools, dark urine, abnormal liver function test (LFT) results, and other metabolic abnormalities.[12] In 90% of those patients who have severe pruritis and metabolic abnormalities resulting from extrahepatic biliary obstruction, percutaneous transhepatic biliary drainage (PTBD) alleviates these conditions.[13,14] Review of patient laboratory data includes a complete blood cell count, coagulation profile, serum urea nitrogen, creatinine, electrolytes, and LFTs, including direct, indirect, and total bilirubin. If there are no signs suggesting biliary sepsis, then intravenous (IV) antibiotics are given the day of the procedure and continued for 24 hours. If a patient presents with signs and symptoms of biliary sepsis, then IV antibiotics are started immediately after blood cultures are obtained.

Patient allergies should be reviewed with prophylaxis given against contrast allergies when indicated. All relevant noninvasive imaging should be reviewed, including ultrasound (US), CT, MRI, and magnetic resonance cholangiopancreatography (MRCP) (**Figs. 1** and **2**). At the authors' institution, patient platelet count is required

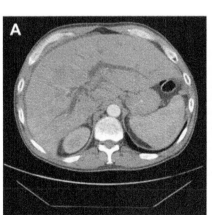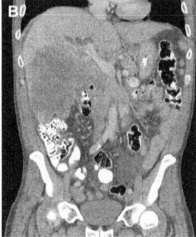

Fig. 1. A 54-year-old man who had unresectable cholangiocarcinoma and biliary obstruction. (*A*) Axial and (*B*) coronal CT images showing biliary ductal dilatation with extensive right lobe and porta hepatis involvement, leading to left-sided approach to drainage.

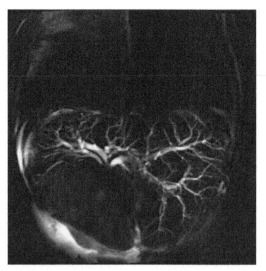

Fig. 2. MRCP showing hilar involvement.

to be greater than 50,000 with transfusion of platelets for levels below 50,000. The international normalized ratio should be less than 1.5, but in patients on warfarin therapy, fresh frozen plasma or vitamin K should be given as determined by the urgency of the procedure. For heparinized patients, the heparin drip can be held 4 hours before the procedure. Subcutaneous heparin injections should be held the morning of the procedure with antiplatelet agents, including aspirin and Plavix (clopidogrel), held 5 days before the procedure. If a patient has undergone recent placement of a drug-eluding coronary stent, however, the situation needs to be discussed with the patient's cardiologist, as withholding these medications could lead to acute thrombosis of the stent.

PREPROCEDURE ANATOMIC EVALUATION AND ACCESS SITE DETERMINATION

With noninvasive imaging techniques continuing to improve, the more invasive percutaneous transhepatic cholangiogram (PTC) as a diagnostic tool has been replaced with CT and MRCP (**Fig. 3**). PTC now is used predominantly as a tool for treatment during PTBD.[15] Patients initially evaluated with noninvasive examinations, such as CT, US, MRI, or MRCP, typically undergo endoscopic retrograde cholangiopancreatography (ERCP) as the next diagnostic tool. This procedure demonstrates excellent biliary and pancreatic duct anatomy and provides for possible biliary decompression.[15] When ERCP fails, PTBD is indicated, especially for more proximal tumors that cannot

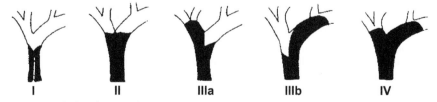

Fig. 3. Bismuth classification. (*From* Cheng JL, Bruno MJ, Bergman JJ, et al. Endoscopic palliation of patients with biliary obstruction caused by nonresectable hilar cholangiocarcinoma: efficacy of self-expandable metallic Wallstents. Gastrointest Endosc 2002;56:33–9; with permission.)

be reached by a transampullary approach. PTC also is preferred for patients who are likely to undergo surgical resection, in which case the biliary drainage catheter often remains in place postoperatively as a stent and as access to the biliary tree. ERCP failure usually is the result of difficult anatomy; complex postoperative anatomy, such as Roux-en-Y diversion or Whipple procedure; tight strictures not allowing for retrograde crossing of the pathology; or cases of bilateral biliary obstruction, which can occur in advanced cases of cholangiocarcinoma.[15,16] Preprocedural evaluation of the biliary tree also allows for determination of whether or not a left or right ductal approach is indicated. Techniques for PTC and drainage are well described,[13,14,17,18] and are accomplished from a subcostal approach into the left duct or an intercostal approach to the right duct system. Advantages of a left subcostal approach include better visualization with sonography, shorter distance to traverse to the left duct system, less catheter pain than intercostal approach, and (in patients who have ascites) less leakage around the catheter.[19]

PERCUTANEOUS TRANSHEPATIC CHOLANGIOGRAPHY

Patients are placed supine with the area of planned access prepped and draped in sterile fashion. If a left-sided approach is planned, then access is accomplished subcostally with a combination of US and fluoroscopic guidance. If a right-sided approach is planned, access is obtained via a mid-right axillary line approach, above the hepatic flexure of the colon. At the authors' institution, dependent on a patient's clinical state and anesthesia availability, conscious sedation or anesthesia provided by the anesthesia team is used. The inferior border of the rib is avoided to prevent injury to the neurovascular bundle. Typically, right-sided access is gained from the 10th rib or inferiorly. More cephalad approaches have increasing risk for traversing the plural space. Fluoroscopy is used to avoid crossing bowel and pleura.[15] At the authors' institution, 21-gauge needle systems (Accustick, Boston Scientific, Natick, Massachusetts) are used. The needle is advanced under fluoroscopic or US guidance into the liver. From a right-sided approach, the needle is passed parallel to the table top with the tip directed medially and superiorly stopping approximately one half to one full vertebral body distance from the lateral margin of the vertebral body itself. The stylet is removed and the needle is connected to a syringe and tubing containing contrast material. The needle is withdrawn slowly with contrast material slowly injected. Once the bile duct is accessed, contrast material flows slowly away from the needle tip confined by a duct or tubular structure. If within a biliary radicle, the contrast material flows toward the hilum or porta hepatis. If the needle is within a branch of the portal vein or hepatic artery, contrast material flows rapidly through the vascular structure toward the periphery of the liver. If it is within the hepatic vein, flow is toward the cardiophrenic angle. Once the needle is within a peripheral aspect of the biliary duct, an over-the-wire exchange for the exchange dilator sheath assembly is made and advanced into the central aspect of the duct system. If a patient has clinical signs of sepsis or the biliary fluid appears dark and viscous or purulent in any way, complete drainage of the biliary tree is performed before diagnostic cholangiography is attempted. If sepsis is suspected, then a bile specimen is sent for microbiologic evaluation. Once drained, contrast material is injected gently with cholangiography images (**Fig. 4**) obtained to define the biliary anatomy. If the initial needle access is too central, then a second 21-gauge needle is used to gain access to a more peripheral duct before placement of the dilator sheath assembly. A peripheral duct access is important as it may decrease the risk for large vessel injury and subsequent morbidity and possibly mortality. Through the outer catheter a 4-French (Fr) Bernstein catheter and wire are

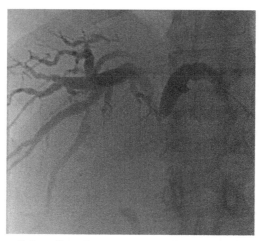

Fig. 4. PTC with Bismuth type III anatomy.

placed coaxially in an attempt to gain access across the obstructive process and allow for placement of an internal/external biliary drainage catheter. Patients usually are placed to external drainage overnight and then the biliary catheter is capped once the clinical scenario of the patient is stable. Nondilated ducts are more difficult to access and, therefore, US may be useful in positioning the needle just anterior to the right portal vein in attempts to improve locating a duct.[15]

TISSUE DIAGNOSIS

If tissue diagnosis still is required when a patient presents for the PTC/PTBD procedure, then cells and tissue can be obtained by several methods. First, bile fluid can be sent for cytology. Second, tissue can be obtained by brush biopsy or (the authors' preferred method) forceps biopsy. Typically an 8-Fr sheath is advanced to the level of the obstruction where coaxially, a myocardial forceps biopsy system is advanced to the edge of the sheath where the forceps are opened and tissue then is obtained. This procedure typically is performed after decompression of the biliary system is performed, particularly in patients who have clinical signs and symptoms of biliary sepsis. This often is done after several days of external drainage to limit the chance of transient bacteremia from the biopsy manipulation.

BILIARY DECOMPRESSION

Once the biliary tree is accessed, review of the cholangiographic anatomy allows for determination of appropriate decompression. Additional drains may be necessary depending on whether or not isolated duct systems are present. If an obstruction cannot be traversed on the initial drainage procedure, an external drainage catheter can be left in place above the obstruction to allow for external decompression. Patients can be brought back after external decompression has been made, oftentimes allowing for crossing of the obstruction with reduction in the inflammation of the biliary system. The goal and management of percutaneous drainage is to re-establish biliary enteric communication and drainage. This can be re-established in one of two ways—percutaneous placement of an internal/external drain versus percutaneous or ERCP placement of internal endoprostheses. These endoprostheses include metallic stents and plastic (silastic) stents. The external drain completely diverts bile outside of the body to a drainage bag. Internal stents (plastic or metal) allow for antegrade flow of bile into the bowel. An internal/external catheter can divert bile to the external bag or allow for internal drainage into the small bowel if capped. The choice of drainage option typically depends on the location of obstruction and whether or not a lesion can be traversed. For patients who are likely to have surgical resection, placement of a permanent metallic stent is contraindicated and only plastic stents should be used unless specifically agreed upon with surgeon.

EXTERNAL BILIARY DRAINAGE

External drainage catheters divert the bile to a drainage bag connected to the drainage catheter. This type of drainage catheter needs to be flushed routinely and routine changes need to be performed at 2- to 3-month intervals. This is to help prevent catheter occlusions and subsequent cholangitis or sepsis. The major disadvantage of external drainage is that with diversion of bile to outside of the body, patients may develop fluid and electrolyte imbalances more commonly than if internal drainage is obtained. Malnutrition also can occur from the lack of bile aiding in digestion and absorption of fat and fat-soluble minerals. In particular, fat malabsorption commonly leads to vitamin K deficiency and resulting coagulopathy. In addition, careful attention by patients and caretakers must be given to preventing catheter dislodgement and infections at the skin site.[3]

INTERNAL/EXTERNAL DRAINAGE CATHETERS

Internal/external drainage catheters allow for internal or external flow of bile depending on whether or not the catheter is capped or uncapped, respectively. The catheter is placed percutaneously as is an external drainage catheter; however, the catheter is longer and contains multiple side holes along the internal aspect proximal to the locking pigtail, which is placed within the small bowel. Thus, once the catheter is capped, antegrade flow of bile can occur as it flows through side holes above the level of obstruction through the catheter lumen and into the small bowel and exits via the side holes within the pigtail of the catheter. This type of drainage is preferred over external drainage as it reduces the issues of fluid and electrolyte imbalances. These catheters also must be changed routinely every 2 to 3 months and often are easier to exchange than internal plastic drains. The disadvantage, however, is that there still is an external portion of the catheter exiting the skin, which is in need of catheter and skin site care.[3]

INTERNAL BILIARY DRAINAGE

Internal biliary drainage is accomplished with metal or plastic stents. These can be placed percutaneously or endoscopically. These stents are placed such that the upper portion of the stent is above the level of obstruction with the distal portion below the obstruction. This allows for bile to flow through the stent and obstruction into the small bowel. A major advantage is that there is no catheter exiting the skin externally to the body. This also allows for enhanced balancing of fluids and electrolytes.[3] Internal stents often are more comfortable, and, because there is no external catheter present to care for, there is no restriction to patients' activities. The major disadvantage of internal stents occurs when a stent becomes occluded or is in need of change or a revision. Plastic endoprostheses are limited by their size and eventual occlusion requiring exchange. Although the median duration of stent patency is 4 months, early occlusion occurs in 6% to 23% of cases.[20,21] The largest inner luminal diameter of the endoscopically placed plastic biliary stent is 3 mm. Larger stents can be placed percutaneously with the sizes ranging from 8 to 12 Fr.[3]

METALLIC STENTS

There are two types of metallic stents used routinely: balloon expandable and self-expanding stents. Self-expanding stents are preferred because of their flexibility and availability in longer lengths. A major drawback of the metal stent is the gaps in the stent wall (called interstices), which can allow for tumor ingrowth and may predispose them to occlusion.[3] There are stents available commercially, however, with a covering or lining (silicone or polytetrafluoroethylene) that may help prevent tumor ingrowth. The stents typically used vary between 8 and 10 mm in diameter. Not only is the larger luminal diameter an advantage but also there is reduced risk for migration. The metal stent should be placed such that the stent covers from above to below the obstructing lesion. If the obstruction is at the level of the hilum, stenting oftentimes is extended into the main right and left ducts in a Y-shaped configuration, to re-establish continuity of the bifurcation (**Fig. 5**). This can aid in antegrade drainage and decrease the risk for cholangitis and septicemia.[22–25] If the obstructing lesion extends further into the biliary tree into second-order biliary radicles or causes isolation of multiple segmental or subsegmental ducts, this technique is not indicated. In this situation, the lobe with greater reserve, less atrophy, and less tumor burden should be considered for plastic stent drainage, allowing for overall improved palliation.[22]

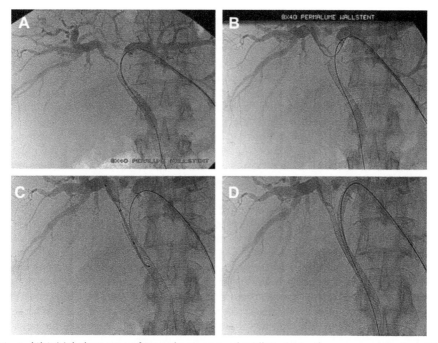

Fig. 5. (*A*) Initial placement of Permalume-covered Wallstent into the common bile duct. (*B*) Catheter crossing over bifurcation from left to right duct. (*C*) Right duct stent being deployed from left access by partially deploying stent in right duct and allowing stent to buckle into the common bile duct by removing wire and advancing delivery system. (*D*) Biliary bifurcation re-established with kissing left and right stents into the common bile duct stent.

GALLBLADDER CARCINOMA

The role of interventional radiologists in the management of gallbladder disease is based on the extent of disease at the time of diagnosis. PTC and drainage usually are reserved for those patients presenting with obstructive jaundice. PTC can aid not only in identifying the level of obstruction but also in offering drainage to relieve an obstruction. The internal/external catheter also may be helpful in surgical management and biliary reconstruction. Generally, however, biliary decompression for gallbladder cancer is used mainly for palliation of unresectable disease. Metallic stents often are used in decompression for unresectable patients.

ADJUNCTIVE THERAPIES

Regarding management of malignant biliary disease, minimally invasive percutaneous methods are not limited to bile duct decompression or tissue diagnosis. Various other procedures are available at many centers, which can be useful as adjunctive therapies to surgical or medical treatments. Transcatheter arterial chemoembolization (TACE), conventional or with drug-eluting beads (DEB), and embolization with yttrium-90–loaded beads are effective methods of delivering regional therapy in patients who have unresectable disease. Additionally, portal vein embolization (PVE) is useful in preoperative management of selected patients before major hepatic resection. An article on this subject by Palavecino, Abdalla, Madoff, and Vauthey appears elsewhere in this issue.

TRANSCATHETER CHEMOEMBOLIZATION AND RADIOEMBOLIZATION

The prognosis for patients who have unresectable intrahepatic cholangiocarcinoma (ICC) is universally poor, with survival lasting 6 to 12 months. Because of the advanced nature of the disease at the time of diagnosis, only approximately 30% of patients are candidates for curative resection.[26–30] Most unresectable patients are candidates for palliative therapies, such as systemic chemotherapy, radiation therapy, or TACE.

TACE, introduced in the 1980s, is based on the concept that hepatic malignancies are preferentially supplied by the hepatic arterial circulation rather than portal flow. Chemotherapeutic agents are delivered through selective arterial catheterization directly to liver tumors in conjunction or followed by an embolic agent.[31–33] The reduction in arterial flow causes some degree of tissue ischemia within the tumor and increases the time for which there is measurable drug activity. As a result, less drug escapes the tumor bed and there are fewer systemic side effects than typically seen with systemic chemotherapy.

Preprocedure evaluation is similar to that for any angiographic procedure. LFTs are obtained to help assess patients' ability to tolerate liver-directed cytotoxic therapy and embolization. TACE is performed via femoral or brachial arterial catheterization. Selective mesenteric arteriography is performed with a 4- or 5-Fr angiographic catheter to identify normal and variant hepatic vascular anatomy, assess portal vein patency, and delineate the arterial supply to the tumor. Selective hepatic arteriography then is performed with a 3- or 4-Fr catheter before treatment. Whenever possible, it is advantageous for the catheter to be positioned as selectively as possible within a tumor's arterial supply before delivering the chemoembolic mixture to minimize damage to normal surrounding liver parenchyma. If disease is widespread throughout the liver, the entire distribution of the right or left hepatic arteries can be treated in a single setting, provided a patient's underlying liver function can tolerate transient ischemia. The opposite lobe then is treated at a later date, typically 4 to 6 weeks after the initial treatment. This allows for the treated lobe to "recuperate" from the previous chemoembolization insult and lessen the risk for complete hepatic failure.

Various protocols for performing TACE are used throughout the world. The most widely used agent worldwide is doxorubicin. In the United States, a combination of cisplatin, doxorubicin, and mitomycin is the preferred drug combination.[34] The combination of drugs is emulsified most often in lipiodol (an iodinated ester derived from poppyseed oil), which acts as a drug carrier and is selectively retained by liver tumors. Delivery of this emulsion usually is followed by particulate embolization with a variety of embolic agents, most frequently polyvinyl alcohol particles (Contour Microspheres, Boston Scientific, Natick, Massachusetts) Embosphere Microspheres (BioSphere Medical, Rockland, Massachusetts) or Gelfoam (Pharmacia & Upjohn, Kalamazoo, Michigan), to reduce the arterial inflow to the tumor and allow for greater contact time of chemotherapy by the tumor.

Serious complications (acute liver failure, liver abscess, tumor rupture, and pulmonary lipiodol embolism) are rare with TACE. The procedure is well tolerated; the most common adverse effect is postembolization syndrome, which consists of varying degrees of abdominal pain, nausea, vomiting, low-grade fever, and elevated LFTs. The syndrome typically is self-limited requiring only symptomatic management and generally resolves in 7 to 10 days.

TACE has been shown to be effective particularly in treatment of unresectable hepatocellular carcinoma (HCC). Prolonged survival in selected patients who have HCC has been demonstrated in two prospective randomized controlled trails.[35,36] Although there are fewer data regarding survival of patients who have ICC treated with TACE, recent data have shown improved survival.[37,38] In addition, there is growing evidence in support of TACE in treatment of unresectable colorectal metastases to the liver,[39–42] as colorectal metastases and ICC demonstrate a similar vascular pattern angiographically.

More recently, there has been increasing interest in the use of DEB as an alternative chemotherapy delivery system. Hydrogel microspheres (LC Beads, AngioDynamics, Queensbury, New York) can be loaded with specific chemotherapeutic agents and delivered intra-arterially in a manner similar to that of conventional TACE. This technique has been growing in favor of conventional TACE in the treatment of HCC with the use of doxorubicin-loaded beads because of an advantageous pharmacokinetic profile, reduced adverse side effects, and improved tumor response by imaging.[43,44] To date, the authors are not aware of any comparative studies between DEB and conventional TACE regarding efficacy in treatment of HCC or ICC. Few data exist regarding the use of DEB in the treatment of ICC but one small study suggests a survival benefit for patients treated with DEB compared with a palliative group.[45,46]

As an alternative to TACE, there is growing interest in radioembolization with yttrium-90 microspheres. Performed in a manner similar to conventional TACE, radioembolization involves the intra-arterial delivery of glass microspheres (SIR Spheres, Sirtex Medical, Wilmington, Massachusetts) and Theraspheres (MDS Nordion, Ottawa, Ontario, Canada) loaded with yttrium-90 directly to hepatic malignancies to promote radiation-induced necrosis. Many studies have demonstrated a positive benefit with respect to progression-free survival, decrease in serum tumor markers, decrease in tumor size on imaging, and decrease in metabolic activity using yttrium-90 microspheres in the treatment of HCC and colorectal liver metastases. Few data exist regarding the efficacy of radioembolization in the treatment of ICC. Conceptually, however, this technique offers a possible treatment alternative to traditional, largely ineffective, systemic therapies for managing cholangiocarcinoma.

PORTAL VEIN EMBOLIZATION

PVE is gaining increasing acceptance for use in patients before surgical resection. PVE usually is reserved for patients whose future liver remnant (FLR) is too small to allow for safe resection. The procedure is safe and effective for inducing selective hypertrophy of nondiseased portions of the liver, thereby decreasing the incidence of postoperative complications and shortening hospital stays. In addition, patients who initially may be considered unresectable because of insufficient hepatic reserve could become surgical candidates after PVE.[47]

A comprehensive understanding of functional liver and portal venous anatomy is critical in performing PVE. A detailed review of normal and variant portal venous anatomy and segmental liver anatomy is beyond the scope of this article. Interventional radiologists performing PVE, however, need to be familiar with this knowledge. Preprocedure evaluation is similar to that for PTC/PTBD regarding laboratory studies and cross-sectional imaging studies.[48]

Several factors need to be considered when deciding whether or not to perform PVE. The FLR to total estimated liver volume (TELV) ratio should be calculated. The presence or absence of underlying liver disease must be considered because this factor determines how much FLR is required for safe resection. A FLR/TELV ratio of at least 25% is recommended for patients who have normal liver and of 40% for patients who have compromised liver function.[49–54] The presence of systemic disease, such as diabetes mellitus, can affect the rate of hypertrophy. Insulin works synergistically with hepatocyte growth factor, which affects the rate of hepatic hypertrophy. There are no absolute contraindications to PVE but relative contraindications include unfavorable location of the tumor, which can preclude safe transhepatic access to the portal vein; tumor invasion of the portal vein; biliary dilatation, which has not been adequately decompressed; uncorrectable coagulopathy; and renal insufficiency.

Broad-spectrum antibiotics should be administered IV on the day of the procedure to minimize the risk for biliary sepsis. As with PTC/PTBD, general anesthesia may be required or requested, but at the authors' institution the procedure typically is performed with moderate sedation (midazolam hydrochloride and fentanyl citrate) and local anesthetic (1% lidocaine hydrochloride). Several factors determine from which side the portal system should be approached. Often, a right-sided approach is preferred because of operator preference, as a left-sided approach can be technically more difficult. Some investigators advocate an ipsilateral approach to the side of the tumor so as not to injure the FLR. A transileocolic venous approach also can be performed at laparotomy.

If a right-sided approach is planned, similar considerations to those for PTC/PTBD are made regarding the pleural space, intercostal neurovascular bundle, and hepatic flexure. At the authors' institution, an Accustick set often is used under fluoroscopic or US guidance to gain access to the portal system. As with PTC/PTBD, access to a peripheral portal vein branch is preferred to minimize the risk for postprocedure bleeding. Seldinger technique then is used to place a 6-Fr vascular sheath into the ipsilateral main right or left portal vein or main portal vein itself. A 5-Fr angiographic pigtail catheter then is placed into the main portal vein where flush portography is performed in multiple obliquities to delineate the portal venous anatomy. If particle embolization is performed, a microcatheter is placed coaxially through a 5-Fr selective angiographic catheter into the segmental branches of the portal vein distribution that is to be embolized. It is the authors' preference to occlude the segmental portal vein branches with Embospheres ranging in size from 300 to 1200 microns in diameter. The smaller particles are used first to occlude the smaller distal branches, followed by the larger particles to occlude the proximal, tertiary branches. Coils or Amplatzer plugs then are used to occlude the first- and second-order portal vein branches. Embolization is performed until stasis or near stasis is achieved (**Fig. 6**). The access tract then is

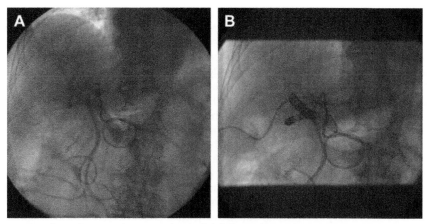

Fig. 6. Transhepatic access into portal vein (*A*) followed by right PVE with coils (*B*).

embolized, usually with Gelfoam, as the sheath is removed. Patients typically are admitted to the hospital for monitoring and symptomatic treatment of postembolization syndrome. Patients are discharged when they are clinically stable and laboratory values are acceptable, usually the next day. A repeat CT scan is performed in approximately 4 weeks to assess FLR hypertrophy and evaluate for progression of disease. If resection is not performed at this time, follow-up CT is performed at monthly intervals. Because an absolute safe FLR volume has yet to be determined, resection typically is performed in patients who demonstrate liver regeneration and whose disease has not progressed significantly.

Complications secondary to PVE are uncommon and are similar to those associated with other transhepatic procedures. These include bleeding (eg, subcapsular hematoma), transient hemobilia, and infection.[47] Portal vein thrombosis and portal hypertension resulting in esophageal varices also can occur rarely. Small bowel obstruction is a complication that rarely occurs but is specific to the transileocolic approach.

COMPLICATIONS AND MANAGEMENT OF PERCUTANEOUS BILIARY INTERVENTIONS

PTC and PTBD are associated with major and minor complications. Once successful percutaneous access to the biliary ductal system is achieved, complications can be seen in acute, subacute, and delayed time frames. During the initial percutaneous access of an obstructed biliary tree, biliary sepsis can occur acutely and manifests as tachycardia, fever, and hypotension. Management should include immediate administration of full antibiotic coverage, IV fluids to support blood pressure, and establishment of adequate external biliary drainage. Close postprocedural observation then is required and may necessitate intensive care monitoring.

Hemobilia occurs in 2.6% to 9% of PTC/PTBD cases.[33] Hemobilia from trauma to the hepatic parenchyma during initial biliary access, or after cholangioplasty/stenting, often is encountered acutely but usually is self-limited and resolves within 48 hours with routine flushing of the biliary catheter. Hemobilia that occurs in a more delayed time frame, sometimes weeks to months postprocedurally, is more serious, and usually indicates the interval development of a hepatic artery pseudoaneurysm. Because this represents arterial communication to the biliary tract, the bleeding can be catastrophic and thus requires immediate intervention. The risk for this occurring is increased with a more central access to the biliary duct during the initial PTC. A temporizing approach to treatment involves upsizing of the biliary catheter (increasing the diameter of the biliary catheter in an attempt to tamponade the pseudoaneurysm). Exchanging the existing catheter over a wire for a larger diameter catheter, however, must be performed carefully and quickly, as excessive bleeding can occur while the existing catheter is removed, as all tamponade effect is lost until the new catheter is in place. If biliary access is lost during the exchange, patients may exsanguinate. At the authors' institution, the preference is to approach hemobilia by making a cholangiographic or angiographic diagnosis, followed by definitive treatment, beginning with a cholangiogram via the biliary catheter, which often shows filling defects within the ducts from residual intraluminal clot but rarely reveals the pseudoaneurysm. An over-the-wire cholangiogram then is performed after the biliary catheter has been exchanged for a same-sized vascular sheath. If the cholangiogram fails to identify the source of bleeding, the authors proceed to hepatic arterial angiography from a femoral artery approach to define the hepatic arterial anatomy. The angiogram often fails to reveal the pseudoaneurysm or source of bleeding while the biliary catheter is in place. With the biliary catheter exchanged for the vascular sheath (which is no longer in the biliary tree), hepatic arteriography is rapidly repeated. If needed, the sheath can be rapidly advanced over-the-wire back into the biliary tree to tamponade the bleed. Review of the arteriogram usually identifies the pseudoaneurysm and its location relative to the biliary ducts. Coil embolization of the pseudoaneurysm then can be performed, which leads to thrombosis of the pseudoaneurysm and resolution of the hemobilia (**Fig. 7**).

Subacute complications generally involve problems with the biliary drainage catheter, biliary stent occlusions, and cholangitis. Drainage catheter problems usually manifest as pericatheter leakage, spontaneously or on flushing of the catheter.

Pericatheter leakage usually indicates that the catheter is occluded distally or that it has migrated proximally, such that a catheter side hole no longer is within the biliary duct but within the hepatic parenchyma, allowing bile or flush to drain retrograde along the catheter tract rather than into the duct. In either case, the diagnosis is made with cholangiography via the catheter, with exchange or repositioning of the catheter as needed.

In the setting of the development of ascites, pericatheter leakage may be secondary to tracking of ascites back up to the entrance of the catheter to the liver edge, where it then exits out the catheter tract. This can be difficult and frustrating to manage, and is treated best with frequent paracentesis if the underlying liver dysfunction cannot be

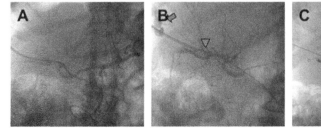

Fig. 7. Hemobilia after right transhepatic biliary drainage. (*A*) Hepatic arteriogram fails to show bleed with biliary catheter in place. (*B*) Marked extravasation (*arrow*) from right hepatic artery injury (*arrowhead*) after catheter removed over wire. (*C*) Successful coil embolization of right hepatic branches ceases bleeding.

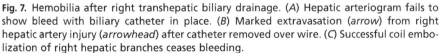

corrected. Alternatively, a purse string suture can be placed around the biliary catheter at insertion site to help "seal" the skin site and prevent continued leakage. Biliary stent occlusions require repeat PTC/PTBD and possibly further cholangioplasty/stenting.

Cholangitis may indicate catheter occlusion or progression of disease such that a ductal segment may have become isolated from the remainder of the biliary tree. Treatment requires antibiotics and re-establishment of adequate biliary drainage via PTC/PTBD. If isolated ducts are present, multiple drainage catheters may be needed to fully decompress the biliary tree.

SUMMARY

Treatment and management of biliary tract malignancies, particularly in inoperable patients, must include percutaneous interventions. These techniques involve direct decompression of biliary obstruction for palliation and vascular approaches to ablate or slow the progression of tumor growth for potential improved quality of life and increased life expectancy. Biliary decompression requires the application of PTC and biliary drainage, cholangioplasty, and stent placement, procedures that generally carry low risk and high probability of success. Vascular interventions include transarterial chemoembolization with various particulate substances that can deliver tumor toxins, such as chemotherapeutic agents or radiation, and direct PVE. PVE encourages hypertrophy of normal hepatic tissue to increase functional liver reserve, which in some instances may transform nonsurgical candidates into surgical candidates for potential resection and cure. In the appropriate patient setting, these vascular interventions are safe and effective. Unfortunately, apart from PVE, these vascular interventions do not yet commonly produce significant increased survivability in patients who have biliary tract malignancies. Continued advances in percutaneous technologies, however, such as those witnessed within the past decade, suggest that future benefits in life expectancy may be achieved.

ACKNOWLEDGMENTS

The authors wish to thank Toni Jones for her assistance in preparing this manuscript.

REFERENCES

1. Nordback IH, Pitt HA, Coleman J, et al. Unresectable hilar cholangiocarcinoma: percutaneous versus operative palliation. Surgery 1994;115:597–603.
2. Pitt HA, Nakeeb A, Abrams RA, et al. Perihilar cholangiocarcinoma: postoperative radiotherapy does not improve survival. Ann Surg 1995;221:788–97.
3. Madoff DC, Wallace MJ. Palliative treatment of unresectable bile duct cancer which stent? Which approach? Surg Oncol Clin N Am 2002;11:923–39.
4. Jarnagin WR. Cholangiocarcinaoma of the extrahepatic bile ducts. Semin Surg Oncol 2000;19:156–76.
5. Henson DE, Albores-Saavedra J, Corle D. Carcinoma of the extrahepatic bile ducts. Histologic types, stage of disease, grade, and survival rates. Cancer 1992;70(6):1498–501.
6. Venbrux AC, Ignacio EA, Soltes AP, et al. Malignant obstruction of the hepatobiliary system. In: Baum SB, Pentecost MJ, editors. (2nd edition) Abram's angiography interventional radiology. Philadelphia: Lippincott; 2006;29:553–9.
7. Clary B, Jarnigan W, Pitt H, et al. Hilar cholangiocarcinoma. J Gastrointest Surg 2004;8(3):298–302.

8. Klatskin G. Adenocarcinoma of the hepatic duct at its bifurcation within the porta hepatis. An unusual tumor with distinctive clinical and pathological features. Am J Med 1965;38:241–56.

9. Available at: www.cholangiocarcinoma.org/definition.htm. 1–2. Accessed May 30, 2008.

10. Craig GR, Peters RL, Edmonson HA. Tumors of the liver and intrahepatic bile ducts. (2nd series). In: Atlas of tumor pathology. Washington, DC: Armed Forces Institute of Pathology; 1989.

11. Dachman AH. Primary biliary neoplasia. In: Friedman AC, Dachman AH, editors. Radiology of the liver biliary tract and pancreas. St. Louis: Mosby; 1994. p. 611–32.

12. Venbrux AC, Osterman FA. Malignant obstruction of the hepatobiliary system. In: Baum SB, Pentecost MJ, editors. Abram's angiography: interventional radiology. Vol III. Philadelphia: Lippincott; 2006;3:472–82.

13. Molnar W, Stockum AE. Relief of obstructive jaundice through percutaneous transhepatic catheter: a new therapeutic method. Am J Roentgenol 1974;122:356–67.

14. Ring EJ, Oleaga JA, Freiman DB, et al. Therapeutic applications of catheter cholangiography. Radiology 1978;128:333–8.

15. Hahn D. Interventional radiology of the gallbladder and biliary tract. In: Gore RM, Levine MS. (3rd edition), Textbook of gastrointestinal radiology. Philadelphia: Saunders; 2008;80:1457–66.

16. Lo SK, Chen J. Role of ERCP in choledocholithiasis. Abdom Imaging 1996;21:120–4.

17. Kaufman SL. Percutaneous biliary drainage for malignant disease. In: Lang EK, Hasso AN, Crues JV III, editors. Biliary radiology. Philadelphia: JB Lippincott, 1992;1:133–42.

18. Mueller PR, vanSonnenberg E, Ferrucci JT Jr. Percutaneous biliary drainage: technical and catheter related problems in 200 procedures. Am J Roentgenol 1982;138:17–23.

19. Koito K, Namieno T, Nagakawa T, et al. Percutaneous transhepatic biliary drainage using color Doppler ultrasonography. J Ultrasound Med 1996;15:203–8.

20. Lammer J, Neumayer K. Biliary drainage endoprostheses: experience with 201 placements. Radiology 1986;159:625–9.

21. Mueller PR, Ferrucci JT Jr, Teplick SK, et al. Biliary stent endoprostheses: analysis of complications in 113 patients. Radiology 1985;156:637–9.

22. Lee MJ, Dawson SL, Mueller PR, et al. Percutaneous management of hilar biliary malignancies with metallic endoprostheses: results, technical problems, and causes of failure. Radiographics 1993;13:1249–63.

23. LaBerge JM, Doherty M, Gordon RL, et al. Hilar malignancy: treatment with an expandable metallic transhepatic biliary stent. Radiology 1990;177:793–7.

24. Gillams A, Dick R, Dooley JS, et al. Self-expandable stainless steel braided endoprosthesis for biliary strictures. Radiology 1990;174:137–40.

25. Lee BH, Choe DH, Lee JH, et al. Metallic stents in malignant biliary obstruction: prospective long-term clinical results. Am J Roentgenol 1997;168:741–5.

26. Chou FF, Sheen-Chen SM, Chen YS, et al. Surgical treatment of cholangiocarcinoma. Hepatogastroenterology 1997;44:760–5.

27. Pitt HA, Grochow LB, Abrams RA. Cancer of the biliary tree. 5th edition. Philadelphia: Lippencott-Raven; 1997.

28. Bismuth H, Castaing D, Traynor O. Resection or palliation: priority of surgery in the treatment of hilar cancer. World J Surg 1988;12:39–47.

29. Burke EC, Jarnagin WR, Hochwald SN, et al. Hilar cholangiocarcinoma: patterns of spread, the importance of hepatic resection for curative operation, and presurgical clinical staging system. Ann Surg 1998;228:385–94.

30. Nakeeb A, Tran KQ, Black MJ, et al. Improved survival in resected biliary malignancies. Surgery 2002;132:555–63.
31. Liapi E, Geschwind JH. Transcatheter and ablative therapeutic approaches for solid malignancies. J Clin Oncol 2007;25:978–86.
32. Yamada R, Nakatsuka H, Nakamura K, et al. Hepatic artery emolization in 32 patients with unresectable hepatoma. Osaka City Med J 1980;26:81–96.
33. Yamada R, Sato M, Kawabata M, et al. Hepatic artery embolization in 120 patients with unresectable hepatoma. Radiology 1983;148:397–401.
34. Hong K, Khwaja A, Liapi E, et al. New intra-arterial drug delivery system for the treatment of liver cancer: preclinical assessment on a rabbit model of liver cancer. Clin Cancer Res 2006;12:2563–7.
35. Lo CM, Ngan H, Tso WK, et al. Randomized controlled trial of transarterial lipiodol chemoembolization for unresectable hepatocellular carcinoma. Hepatology 2002;35:1164–71.
36. Llovet JM, Real MI, Montana X, et al. Arterial embolisation or chemoembolisation versus symptomatic treatment in patients with unresectable hepatocellular carcinoma: a randomized controlled trial. Lancet 2002;359:1734–9.
37. Burger I, Hong K, Schulick R, et al. Transcatheter arterial chemoembolization in unresectable cholangiocarcinoma: initial experience at a single institution. J Vasc Interv Radiol 2005;16:353–61.
38. Kim JH, Yoon H, Sung K, et al. Transcatheter arterial chemoembolization or chemoinfusion for unresectable intrahepatic cholangiocarcinoma. Cancer 2008;113: 1614–22.
39. Lang EK, Brown CL Jr. Colorectal metastases to the liver: selective chemoembolization. Radiology 1993;189:417–22.
40. Martinelly DJ, Wadler S, Bakal CW, et al. Utility of embolization of chemoembolization as second-line treatment in patients with advanced or recurrent colorectal carcinoma. Cancer 1994;74:1706–12.
41. Abramson RJ, Rosen MP, Perry LJ, et al. Cost-effectiveness of hepatic artery chemoembolization for colorectal liver metastases refractory to systemic chemotherapy. Radiology 2000;216:485–91.
42. Salman HS, Cynamon J, Jagust M, et al. Randomized phase II trial of embolization therapy versus chemoembolization therapy in previously treated patients with colorectal carcinoma metastatic to the liver. Clin Colorectal Cancer 2002;2:173–9.
43. Varela M, Real MI, Burrel M, et al. Chemoembolization of hepatocellular with drug eluting beads: efficacy and doxorubicin pharmacokinetics. J Hepatol 2006;46: 474–81.
44. Cobstantin M, Funueanu G, Bortolotti F, et al. Preparation and characterisation of poly(vinyl alcohol)/cyclodextrin microsphers as matrix for inclusion and separation of drugs. Int J Pharm 2004;285:87–96.
45. Aliberti C, Benea G, Massimo T, et al. Chemoembolization (TACE) of unresectable intrahepatic cholangiocarcinoma with slow-release doxorubicin-eluting beads: preliminary results. Cardiovasc Intervent Radiol 2007;31:883–8.
46. Salem R, Thurston KG. Radioembolization with yttrium-90 microspheres: a state-of-the-art brachytherapy treatment for primary and secondary liver malignancies: part 3: comprehensive literature review and future direction. J Vasc Interv Radiol 2006;17:1571–93.
47. Madoff DC, Hick ME, Abdalla EK, et al. Portal vein embolization using polyvinyl alcohol particles and coils in preparation for major liver resection for hepatobiliary malignancy: safety and efficacy—a study in 25 patients. Radiology 2003;227: 251–60.

48. Madoff DC, Hicks ME, Vauthey JN, et al. Transhepatic portal vein embolization: anatomy, indications and technical considerations. Radiographics 2002;22:1063–76.
49. Vauthey JN, Chaoui A, Do KA, et al. Standardized measurement of the future liver remnant prior to extended liver resection: methodology and clinical associations. Surgery 2000;127:512–9.
50. Abdalla EK, Hick ME, Vauthey JN. Portal vein embolization: rationale, technique and future prospects. Br J Surg 2001;88:165–75.
51. Shimamura T, Nakajima Y, Une Y, et al. Efficacy and safety of preoperative percutaneous transhepatic portal vein embolization with absolute ethanol: a clinical study. Surgery 1997;121:135–41.
52. Lee KC, Kinoshita H, Hirohashi K, et al. Extension of surgical indication for hepatocellular carcinoma by portal vein embolization. World J Surg 1993;17:109–15.
53. Kubota K, Makuuchi M, Kusaka K, et al. Measurement of liver volume and hepatic functional reserve as a guide to decision-making in resectional surgery for hepatic tumors. Hepatology 1997;26:1176–81.
54. Azoulay D, Castaing D, Krissat J, et al. Percutaneous portal vein portal vein embolization increases the feasibility and safety of major liver resection for hepatocellular carcinoma in injured liver. Ann Surg 2000;232:665–72.

Portal Vein Embolization in Hilar Cholangiocarcinoma

Martin Palavecino, MD[a], Eddie K. Abdalla, MD[a], David C. Madoff, MD[b],
Jean-Nicolas Vauthey, MD[a],*

KEYWORDS

• Portal vein • Embolization • Hilar cholangiocarcinoma

Various types of liver resection in combination with extrahepatic bile duct resection have been proposed for the treatment of hilar cholangiocarcinoma. In selecting the type of resection, anatomic and oncologic features must be considered. Anatomically, Couinaud[1] showed that although there are biliary variations of hepatic duct confluence with the common bile duct, the left hepatic duct is present in 97% of patients (**Fig. 1**). In addition, the left bile duct is mostly extrahepatic, located strategically at the base of segment 4 and extends to the left for a length of 1 to 5 cm.[1] These characteristics aid in the extension of the resection toward the left, away from the biliary confluence, while minimizing the likelihood of positive margins and facilitating the biliary reconstruction.

For these reasons, at The University of Texas M. D. Anderson Cancer Center, an extended right hepatectomy is favored in most patients with hilar cholangiocarcinoma. According to the Bismuth-Corlette[2] classification, for types I, II, and IIIa hilar cholangiocarcinoma, an extended right hepatectomy is usually performed, whereas for type IIIb hilar cholangiocarcinoma, a left or extended left hepatectomy is performed (**Fig. 2**). In both surgical approaches, segment 4 must be completely or partially resected because most hilar cholangiocarcinomas extend to involve the base of segment 4. The authors do not recommend isolated bile duct resections or central resections for these tumors because of the limited margins and multiple bile duct anastomoses, both of which increase the risk of bile leaks and recurrences.

Patients with proximal bile duct carcinomas are more likely to have postoperative liver dysfunction because of the extensive resection of nontumorous liver necessary

Jean-Nicolas Vauthey, MD, is a consultant for Sanofi-aventis and Genentech. Dr. Vauthey received honoraria from sanofi-aventis and Genentech. Drs. Vauthey and Abdalla have received research funding from Sanofi-aventis.
[a] Department of Surgical Oncology, The University of Texas M. D. Anderson Cancer Center, 1515 Holcombe Boulevard, Unit 444, Houston, TX 77030, USA
[b] Department of Diagnostic Radiology, The University of Texas M. D. Anderson Cancer Center, Houston, TX, USA
* Corresponding author.
E-mail address: jvauthey@mdanderson.org (J-N. Vauthey).

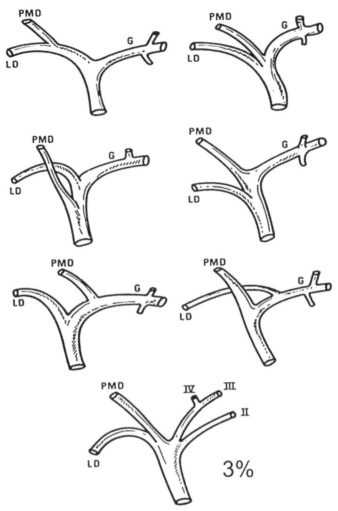

Fig. 1. Variations in biliary anatomy. The left hepatic duct is long and present in 97% of patients. In types I, II, and IIIa hilar cholangiocarcinomas, an extended right hepatectomy permits placement of a safe and single anastomosis away from the confluence, minimizing the probability of positive margins. G, left; LD, lateral right; PMD, para-medial right. (*From* Couinaud C. Le foie. Etudes anatomiques et chirurgicales. Paris: Masson; 1957. p. 469–79; with permission.)

to achieve an oncologically adequate liver resection. To overcome this problem, portal vein embolization (PVE) has been increasingly used before resection. Makuuchi and colleagues[3,4] proposed PVE as a means to produce hypertrophy of the future liver remnant, decreasing the rate of postoperative liver dysfunction after extended liver resections. This procedure was proposed after it was observed that liver dysfunction did not occur in patients undergoing extended resections for hilar cholangiocarcinoma occluding a branch of the portal vein. In 1990, Makuuchi and colleagues[4] published an article about the initial experience with PVE in 14 patients with hilar biliary tract carcinoma. Since that publication, the number of reports on PVE in patients with cholangiocarcinoma has increased yearly.

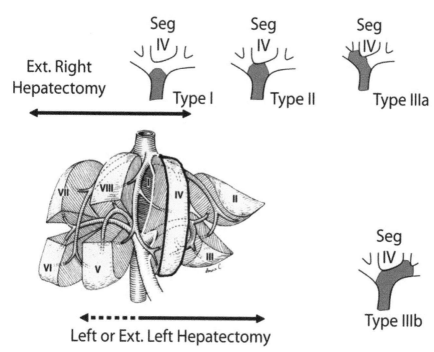

Fig. 2. Extent of hepatic resection according to Bismuth-Corlette classification of hilar chol-angiocarcinoma. (*Adapted from* Parikh AA, Abdalla EK, Vauthey JN. Operative consider-ations in resection of hilar cholangiocarcinoma. HPB 2005;7:254–8; with permission.)

TECHNIQUE
Approach

PVE can be performed by two different approaches: transileocolic and transhe-patic.[5–8] The transileocolic approach is performed intraoperatively by introducing a catheter in the ileocolic vein and embolizing all the portal branches to be resected. It is important to embolize all branches to avoid recanalization of the portal vein by portal-portal shunts. Indications for this approach include the preference of the surgical group, the lack of availability of a radiologic team with skills in percutaneous liver procedures, and the percutaneous approach being infeasible. The advantage of the transileocolic approach is the ability to assess the extent of disease during the same procedure (eg, involvement of adjacent structures, peritoneal disease, and lymph node metastases). The disadvantages are the necessity for general anesthesia and the potential complications caused by the associated laparotomy.

The transhepatic procedure can be performed by an ipsilateral or contralateral approach. The ipsilateral approach was described by Nagino and colleagues[9] from the University Graduate School of Medicine, Nagoya, Japan. This is the preferred approach in the authors' group.[6,10,11] When an extended right hepatectomy is neces-sary, the right PVE should be extended to segment 4 to achieve a better degree of hypertrophy of the future liver remnant and minimize likelihood of tumor growth.[12,13] A peripheral branch of the portal vein to be resected is approached percutaneously. A standard angiographic catheter for combined particulate and coil embolization is used. Segment 4 is embolized first, and a reverse-curved catheter is used to complete the right PVE. The access tract is embolized to reduce the risk of hemorrhage. The main advantages of the ipsilateral approach are the use of standard angiographic catheters and preservation of the future liver remnant by puncturing the ipsilateral hemiliver. The disadvantage is the difficulty in performing the puncture when tumors are large (ie, potential for tumor transgression during puncture). By contrast, the contralateral approach is the most widespread technique for PVE. It was first described by Kinoshita and colleagues.[14] The advantage of this technique is its simplicity because of the straight access to the right portal vein from the left portal vein. The disadvantages are the risk of injury to the future liver remnant, the prolonged time the catheter may remain within the left portal vein that may lead to thrombus formation along the catheter and possibly lead to left portal vein thrombosis. Further, segment 4 embolization, if needed, may prove difficult secondary to the location and angulation of the segment 4 portal veins from left portal vein.

Different embolic materials have been used for PVE, including a mixture of gelatin sponge cubes or powder, diatrizoate sodium meglumine, and gentamicin;[3,4,7] fibrin glue mixed with iodized oil;[9] absolute ethanol;[15] polyvinyl alcohol particles,[6] tris-acryl gelatin microspheres[16] and n-butyl cyanoacrylate.[17,18] No significant differences were found between rates of hypertrophy when different materials were used.[10] The differences among the various embolic materials have been described elsewhere.[6]

Embolization of Segment 4

In the treatment of cholangiocarcinoma, extended right hepatectomy usually with segment 1 resection is needed for curative resection.[4,12] Sufficient volume of remaining segments 2 and 3 is important to minimize the risk of postoperative complications. An adequate future liver remnant is associated with improved liver function after resection as measured by bilirubin clearance[19] and indocyanine green excretion.[20] In addition, in a previous study the authors demonstrated a negative correlation between the future liver remnant volume and the postoperative peak values of alkaline phosphatase level, prothrombin time, and bilirubin clearance.[21] Before an extended right hepatectomy, the surgeon needs to maximize the hypertrophy of the future liver remnant.

Embolization of the portal vein branch of segment 4 is controversial: the technique was first described by Nagino and colleagues[12] who proposed its use to increase the hypertrophy of segments 2 and 3. Other authors, however, have reported the same degree of hypertrophy whether or not segment 4 is embolized; they recommend performing only right PVE even before extended right hepatectomies.[22,23]

The authors recommend embolization of segment 4 before an extended right hepatectomy because they found increased hypertrophy in segments 2 and 3 after right PVE that included segment 4 branches.[13] In their study, the volume of segments 2 and 3 increased by 54% in the group that had segment 4 embolized compared with only 26% in the group that did not have segment 4 embolized ($P = .021$). Despite the greater theoretical possibility of migration of the embolization material to segments 2 and 3 when segment 4 is also embolized,[22] they found a similar rate of coil migration in both groups.[13]

INDICATIONS

Different factors should be taken into account before PVE is performed.

Underlying Liver Function

Patients with biliary tract cancers usually present with obstructive jaundice. Biliary decompression of the future liver remnant before PVE is mandatory to improve liver function and allow the future liver remnant to hypertrophy. Decompression of the future liver remnant should be performed using the unilateral approach, even in patients without communication between the right and left hepatic ducts.[5] Bilateral decompression should be performed in patients with persistent cholangitis after unilateral drainage and in patients with persistent elevation of the bilirubin after unilateral drainage.[24]

Future Liver Remnant

In a study of 102 Western patients without liver disease, the authors found that the right liver accounts for two thirds and the left liver for one third of the total liver volume. There are marked variations, however, in intrahepatic volumetric distribution. Segments 2 and 3 represent approximately 16% of the total liver volume (range, 5%–27%), and in more than 75% of patients the two segments together represent less than 20% of the total liver volume (**Fig. 3**).[25] To avoid liver dysfunction, the volume of the future liver remnant must be considered according to the patient's size. To avoid unnecessary PVE, precise measurement of the future liver remnant is mandatory, given interpatient variation.

The future liver remnant can be assessed using three-dimensional contrast-enhanced CT. Briefly, the contours of the future liver remnant are delineated on the screen, and volume is calculated by adding each slice's volume, determined by the surface area, slice thickness, and space between slices.[26] The three-dimensional reconstruction is accurate; the error associated with this measurement is less than 5%.[27]

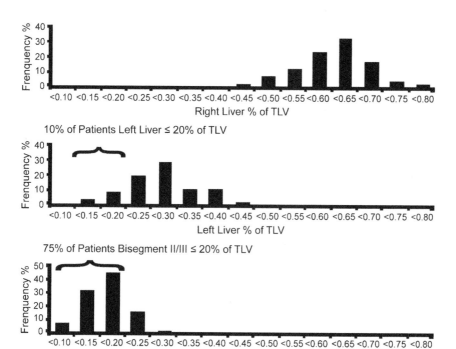

Fig. 3. Volumetric variability of the right liver, left liver, and segments 2 and 3. On average, the right liver (segments 5–8) constitutes two thirds of the total liver volume (TLV), and the left liver (segments 2–4) one third. The left lateral section constitutes 16% of the TLV (range, 5%–27%); in more than 75% of patients, it constitutes less than or equal to 20%. (*Adapted from* Abdalla EK, Denys A, Chevalier P, et al. Total and segmental variations: implications for liver surgery. Surgery 2004;135:404–10; with permission.)

Total liver volume can be estimated using the same technique as that described for the future liver remnant. This measurement could be inaccurate, however, for several reasons. In patients with large or multifocal tumors, the tumor volume needs to be subtracted from the total liver volume. This increases the time required for calculation and the possibility of error.[27] In patients with cholangiocarcinoma, the total liver volume can be overestimated because of extensive biliary dilatation. In cirrhotic patients with enlarged or shrunken liver, the volume is also inaccurate.

To overcome these issues, the authors determined a formula based on body surface area.[26] Body surface area and weight have a linear correlation with liver volume,[21,26,28] and this correlation has been used to calculate liver graft size in living donor liver transplantation.[29] The estimated liver volume is calculated using the following formula:

Total liver volume $= -794.41 + 1267.28 \times$ body surface area

This formula was determined using data from patients from Europe and the United States, and it has been validated by a meta-analysis comparing 12 different formulas.[30]

The standardized future liver remnant (standardized future liver remnant = future liver remnant/estimated total liver volume) can be used to determine whether PVE is indicated.[27] In normal livers, if the standardized future liver remnant is less than or equal to 20% of total liver volume, PVE should be considered. This cutoff has been validated in 66 patients undergoing resection in whom complication rates (any complications, major complications, liver-related complications, hepatic dysfunction, and hepatic insufficiency) were significantly lower when the standardized future liver remnant was greater than 20% of total liver volume.[31] In patients who received extensive chemotherapy, preoperative PVE should be considered when the standardized future liver remnant is less than or equal to 30% of total liver volume.[32] In patients with cirrhosis, PVE should be performed when the standardized future liver remnant is less than or equal to 40% of total liver volume.

After PVE, the future liver remnant volume increases during the first 3 weeks; 75% of the growth of the future liver remnant occurs between days 1 and 21. Subsequently, the hypertrophy reaches a plateau period, with minimal regeneration between days 21 and 56. This plateau period represents a steady-state phase of liver growth during which the future liver remnant after PVE should be evaluated. Patients with insufficient

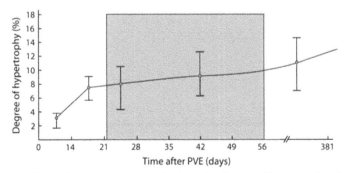

Fig. 4. Kinetics of future liver remnant growth, plotted as degree of hypertrophy after PVE. The shaded zone indicates the period without significative changes between measurement points. (*Adapted from* Ribero D, Abdalla EK, Madoff DC, et al. Portal vein embolization before major hepatectomy and its effects on regeneration, resectability and outcome. Br J Surg 2007;94:1386–94; with permission.)

hypertrophy 3 weeks after PVE are unlikely to develop further hypertrophy beyond this point. Post-PVE imaging performed before 3 weeks may underestimate the degree of hypertrophy (**Fig. 4**).[31]

In the authors' previous study,[31] a degree of hypertrophy (degree of hypertrophy = standardized future liver remnant post-PVE - standardized future liver remnant pre-PVE) less than or equal to 5% predicted the occurrence of postoperative complications in general, liver-related complications, and liver dysfunction. Combining the cutoffs (standardized future liver volume >20% and degree of hypertrophy >5%), liver dysfunction was predicted with a sensitivity of 80%, a specificity of 94%, a positive predictive value of 80%, and a negative predictive value of 94%.[31]

PVE is a safe procedure, but it has contraindications. These include severe coagulopathy; tumoral extension into the future liver remnant; portal hypertension (the authors recommend measurement of portal pressure before embolization); and biliary obstruction in the future liver remnant (an ipsilateral biliary drainage should be performed).

COMPLICATIONS

As with other hepatic percutaneous procedures, PVE is associated with different complications, such as subcapsular hematoma, hemoperitoneum, pseudoaneurysm, portal vein thrombosis, pneumothorax, and infection. In the largest series (240 patients) describing PVE for the treatment of biliary cancers, Nagino and colleagues[33] reported only two major complications: one case of hypersplenism with splenomegaly successfully resected, and one extensive portal and mesenteric vein thrombosis unresected because of locally advanced cancer. In the authors' series of 112 PVEs,[31] eight patients (9%) had PVE-related major complications: four partial portal thromboses (one treated with anticoagulant therapy, two removed surgically, and one left untreated because of systemic progression of disease); one complete portal vein thrombosis (treated with local infusion of recombinant tissue plasminogen activator); one subcapsular hematoma; one esophageal hemorrhage; and one migration of coils (successfully resected).

Such symptoms as pain, fever, nausea, and vomiting are rare. Total bilirubin levels may be increased, as may be prothrombin time. These increased values usually return to pre-PVE levels within 7 to 10 days of surgery.[5,34] Aspartate transaminase and alanine transaminase levels usually do not increase.

The systematic measurement of portal pressure is advocated before PVE to avoid embolizing patients with occult portal hypertension. The authors have used the ipsilateral approach to minimize the risk of injury to the future liver remnant. PVE can be a safe procedure with minimum complications if it is performed by a trained team with close interaction among its members.

OUTCOMES

PVE improves resectability and prevents postoperative hepatic dysfunction in patients with biliary tract cancers whose future liver remnant before extended hepatectomy is expected to be of inadequate size. PVE achieves this improvement without impairing postoperative outcome and survival.

In a recent meta-analysis, Abulkhir and colleagues[34] examined 37 publications including 1088 patients who underwent PVE before liver resection for liver tumors. Cholangiocarcinoma was the primary tumor in 430 patients (39%). There was no mortality related to PVE. After resection, the overall mortality and morbidity rates for the whole series were 1.7% and 16%, respectively.

In the series by Nagino and colleagues[33] liver resection was possible in 80.4% of 240 patients with biliary tract cancer who underwent PVE. The overall mortality rate for the whole series was 8.8%. The mortality rate improved to 4.8%, however, when they analyzed the last 4 years of the study. This mortality rate is similar to that reported for patients who did not undergo preoperative PVE, even when the surgical procedures were less complex. The 1-, 3-, and 5-year survival rates for patients with cholangiocarcinoma who underwent surgical resection were 67%, 42%, and 27% with preoperative PVE and 70%, 43%, and 28% without preoperative PVE ($P =$ NS).

Between 1984 and 2005, at M. D. Anderson Cancer Center, 65 patients underwent resection for extrahepatic bile duct adenocarcinoma, including 36 patients with hilar cholangiocarcinoma. PVE was selectively performed in patients with a future liver remnant less than or equal to 20% of the total estimated liver volume (**Fig. 5**). Perioperative mortality was 4% and the morbidity was 66%. Overall survival and locoregional recurrence rates were compared between patients with R0 resections and patients with a high risk of locoregional recurrence (R1 resection or positive nodes)

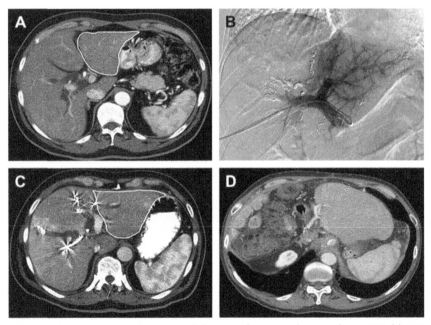

Fig. 5. Scans from a 64-year-old man with history of nausea, decreased appetite, bloating, early satiety, and jaundice. Cholangio MRI revealed bilateral bile duct dilatation with an abrupt interruption at the biliary confluence. Endoscopic retrograde cholangiopancreatography (ERCP) was performed, and brush cytology revealed malignant cells. A stent was placed in the left hepatic duct. (*A*) Post-ERCP CT scan showed dilatation of the right hepatic duct and poststent improvement of the left hepatic duct dilatation. The standardized future liver remnant (segments 2 and 3) was 19% of total liver volume. (*B*) Right PVE extended to segment 4 portal branches was indicated. (*C*) A CT scan performed 4 weeks after PVE showed vascular changes in the right liver with hypertrophy of segments 2 and 3 (the post-PVE standardized future liver remnant was 26% of total liver volume). An extended right hepatectomy with segment 1 resection was performed. An abutment of the left portal vein was found, and a partial left portal vein resection was performed. (*D*) The 3-year follow-up CT scan showed no evidence of disease.

who received adjuvant chemoradiation. With a median follow-up of 31 months, both groups had a similar 5-year overall survival rate (36% versus 42%; $P = .6$) and locoregional recurrence rate (38% versus 37%; $P = .13$).[35]

SUMMARY

The only potentially curative treatment for biliary tract cancer is surgery. Extended right hepatectomy and caudate lobe resection is often performed to achieve a R0 resection. To minimize the risk of postoperative liver dysfunction, in patients with an estimated future liver remnant less than or equal to 20% PVE should be performed. If after PVE the estimated future liver remnant is less than or equal to 20% or the degree of hypertrophy is less than or equal to 5%, liver resection is considered a high-risk procedure and may be contraindicated. If the patient has biliary dilatation of the future liver remnant, a biliary drainage catheter should be placed before PVE. After portal pressure has been measured, the authors prefer to perform PVE using the ipsilateral approach. If the planned surgery is an extended right hepatectomy, segment 4 branch embolization improves the hypertrophy of segments 2 and 3. In high-volume centers with experience in the management of liver malignancies, PVE can be safely performed. PVE increases the resectability rate, and patients who undergo resection with PVE achieve the same overall survival rate as those who undergo resection without PVE.

REFERENCES

1. Couinaud C. Le Foie. Etudes anatomiques et chirurgicales. Paris: Masson; 1957. p. 469–79 [In French].
2. Bismuth H, Corlette MB. Intrahepatic cholangioenteric anastomosis in carcinoma of the hilus of the liver. Surg Gynecol Obstet 1975;140(2):170–8.
3. Makuuchi M, Takayasu K, Takuma T, et al. Preoperative transcatheter embolization of the portal venous branch for patients receiving extended lobectomy due to the bile duct carcinoma. J Jpn Soc Clin Surg 1984;45:1558–64.
4. Makuuchi M, Thai BL, Takayasu K, et al. Preoperative portal embolization to increase safety of major hepatectomy for hilar bile duct carcinoma: a preliminary report. Surgery 1990;107(5):521–7.
5. Imamura H, Takayama T, Makuuchi M. Place of portal vein embolization. In: Blumgart L, editor. Surgery of the liver, biliary tract, and pancreas, vol 2. Philadelphia: Saunders Elsevier; 2006. p. 1452–60.
6. Madoff DC, Abdalla EK, Vauthey JN. Portal vein embolization in preparation for major hepatic resection: evolution of a new standard of care. J Vasc Interv Radiol 2005;16(6):779–90.
7. Imamura H, Shimada R, Kubota M, et al. Preoperative portal vein embolization: an audit of 84 patients. Hepatology 1999;29(4):1099–105.
8. Vauthey JN, Madoff DC, Abdalla EK. Preoperative portal vein embolization: a Western perspective. In: Blumgart LH, editor. Surgery of the liver, biliary tract, and pancreas, vol 2. Philadelphia: Saunders Elsevier; 2006. p. 1461–71.
9. Nagino M, Nimura Y, Kamiya J, et al. Selective percutaneous transhepatic embolization of the portal vein in preparation for extensive liver resection: the ipsilateral approach. Radiology 1996;200(2):559–63.
10. Abdalla EK, Hicks ME, Vauthey JN. Portal vein embolization: rationale, technique and future prospects. Br J Surg 2001;88(2):165–75.
11. Vauthey JN, Pawlik TM, Abdalla EK, et al. Is extended hepatectomy for hepatobiliary malignancy justified? Ann Surg 2004;239(5):722–30.

12. Nagino M, Kamiya J, Kanai M, et al. Right trisegment portal vein embolization for biliary tract carcinoma: technique and clinical utility. Surgery 2000;127(2):155–60.
13. Kishi Y, Madoff DC, Abdalla EK, et al. Is embolization of segment 4 portal veins prior to extended right hepatectomy justified? Surgery 2008;144(5):744–51.
14. Kinoshita H, Sakai K, Hirohashi K, et al. Preoperative portal vein embolization for hepatocellular carcinoma. World J Surg 1986;10(5):803–8.
15. Shimamura T, Nakajima Y, Une Y, et al. Efficacy and safety of preoperative percutaneous transhepatic portal embolization with absolute ethanol: a clinical study. Surgery 1997;121(2):135–41.
16. Madoff DC, Abdalla EK, Gupta S, et al. Transhepatic ipsilateral right portal vein embolization extended to segment IV: improving hypertrophy and resection outcomes with spherical particles and coils. J Vasc Interv Radiol 2005;16(2 Pt 1): 215–25.
17. Denys A, Lacombe C, Schneider F, et al. Portal vein embolization with N-butyl cyanoacrylate before partial hepatectomy in patients with hepatocellular carcinoma and underlying cirrhosis or advanced fibrosis. J Vasc Interv Radiol 2005; 16(12):1667–74.
18. Di Stefano DR, de Baere T, Denys A, et al. Preoperative percutaneous portal vein embolization: evaluation of adverse events in 188 patients. Radiology 2005; 234(2):625–30.
19. Ijichi M, Makuuchi M, Imamura H, et al. Portal embolization relieves persistent jaundice after complete biliary drainage. Surgery 2001;130(1):116–8.
20. Uesaka K, Nimura Y, Nagino M. Changes in hepatic lobar function after right portal vein embolization: an appraisal by biliary indocyanine green excretion. Ann Surg 1996;223(1):77–83.
21. Vauthey JN, Chaoui A, Do KA, et al. Standardized measurement of the future liver remnant prior to extended liver resection: methodology and clinical associations. Surgery 2000;127(5):512–9.
22. Capussotti L, Muratore A, Ferrero A, et al. Extension of right portal vein embolization to segment IV portal branches. Arch Surg 2005;140(11):1100–3.
23. Farges O, Belghiti J, Kianmanesh R, et al. Portal vein embolization before right hepatectomy: prospective clinical trial. Ann Surg 2003;237(2):208–17.
24. Nagino M, Takada T, Miyazaki M, et al. Preoperative biliary drainage for biliary tract and ampullary carcinomas. J Hepatobiliary Pancreat Surg 2008;15(1): 25–30.
25. Abdalla EK, Denys A, Chevalier P, et al. Total and segmental liver volume variations: implications for liver surgery. Surgery 2004;135(4):404–10.
26. Vauthey JN, Abdalla EK, Doherty DA, et al. Body surface area and body weight predict total liver volume in Western adults. Liver Transpl 2002;8(3):233–40.
27. Abdalla EK, Barnett CC, Doherty D, et al. Extended hepatectomy in patients with hepatobiliary malignancies with and without preoperative portal vein embolization. Arch Surg 2002;137(6):675–80.
28. Urata K, Kawasaki S, Matsunami H, et al. Calculation of child and adult standard liver volume for liver transplantation. Hepatology 1995;21(5):1317–21.
29. Nishizaki T, Ikegami T, Hiroshige S, et al. Small graft for living donor liver transplantation. Ann Surg 2001;233(4):575–80.
30. Johnson TN, Tucker GT, Tanner MS, et al. Changes in liver volume from birth to adulthood: a meta-analysis. Liver Transpl 2005;11(12):1481–93.
31. Ribero D, Abdalla EK, Madoff DC, et al. Portal vein embolization before major hepatectomy and its effects on regeneration, resectability and outcome. Br J Surg 2007;94(11):1386–94.

32. Adam R, Delvart V, Pascal G, et al. Rescue surgery for unresectable colorectal liver metastases downstaged by chemotherapy: a model to predict long-term survival. Ann Surg 2004;240(4):644–57 [discussion 657–8].
33. Nagino M, Kamiya J, Nishio H, et al. Two hundred forty consecutive portal vein embolizations before extended hepatectomy for biliary cancer: surgical outcome and long-term follow-up. Ann Surg 2006;243(3):364–72.
34. Abulkhir A, Limongelli P, Healey AJ, et al. Preoperative portal vein embolization for major liver resection: a meta-analysis. Ann Surg 2008;247(1):49–57.
35. Borghero Y, Crane CH, Szklaruk J, et al. Extrahepatic bile duct adenocarcinoma: patients at high-risk for local recurrence treated with surgery and adjuvant chemoradiation have an equivalent overall survival to patients with standard-risk treated with surgery alone. Ann Surg Oncol 2008;15(11):3147–56.

Extrahepatic Cholangiocarcinoma: Current Surgical Strategy

Cherif Boutros, MD, MSc, Ponnandai Somasundar, MD,
N. Joseph Espat, MD, MS*

KEYWORDS

• Cholangiocarcinoma • Distal • Extrahepatic • Surgery

Cholangiocarcinoma (CCA) is a rare cancer; overall, the annual incidence is approximately 1 per 100,000 in the United States; 5.5 per 100,000 in Japan; 6.5 per 100,000 among American Indians; and 7.3 per 100,000 in Israel.[1] Although rare, it remains the second most common hepatobiliary cancer and its incidence is increasing worldwide[2] likely because of improvement in diagnosis and better knowledge of the natural history of the disease.[3] Extrahepatic CCA can occur anywhere along the biliary tree and prognosis varies according to the location of disease.

Extrahepatic CCA is defined as cancer arising from the common bile duct, the hepatic duct bifurcation, or the first-order left and right hepatic ducts. Extrahepatic CCA can be subdivided as distal (or intrapancreatic) CCA, arising from the intrapancreatic portion of the common bile duct, and proximal/hilar CCA, which arises at the level of the hepatic duct bifurcation and first-order hepatic ducts.

CLASSIFICATION

Various classification schemes have been proposed for extrahepatic CCA. According to the Japanese Society of Biliary Surgery, extrahepatic CCA is classified according to its location as (1) portal (hilar), which is at or above the confluence (bifurcation) of the common hepatic duct; (2) superior, which is between the hepatic duct confluence and the cystic duct-hepatic duct junction; (3) middle, which is located in between the cystic duct-hepatic duct junction and the pancreatic segment of the bile duct; and (4) distal bile duct, which travels from the superior border of the pancreas to its entrance into the duodenal wall.[4]

Department of Hepatobiliary and Surgical Oncology, Roger Williams Medical Center, Boston University School of Medicine, 825 Chalkstone Avenue, Prior 4, Providence, RI 02908, USA
* Corresponding author. Roger Williams Medical Center, Boston University School of Medicine, 825 Chalkstone Avenue, Prior 4, Providence, RI 02908, USA.
E-mail address: jespat@hepaticsurgery.com (N.J. Espat).

Surg Oncol Clin N Am 18 (2009) 269–288
doi:10.1016/j.soc.2008.12.003
1055-3207/08/$ – see front matter © 2009 Elsevier Inc. All rights reserved.

surgonc.theclinics.com

In another simpler classification scheme, Nakeeb and collegues[5] classified CCA into three categories: intrahepatic, perihilar, and distal. The distal group includes those located in the extrahepatic bile duct distal to the hepatic duct bifurcation, including the intrapancreatic bile duct tumors. The distal type is the second most common (27%) after the perihilar type (67%). Tumors of the hepatic duct bifurcation are classified into four types according to the Bismuth classification:[6] type I, CCA of the common hepatic duct; type II, involvement of the hepatic duct bifurcation; type IIIA, tumor extending to the right hepatic duct; type IIIB, tumor extending to the left hepatic duct; and type IV, tumor extending to both right and left hepatic ducts.

Another classification based on tumor morphology and growth pattern, proposed by Lim and Park,[7] describes three different categories: mass forming (nodular), periductal infiltrating, and intraductal growing.

In this article, two groups (sites) of extrahepatic CCA are discussed separately: hilar and middle-distal origin disease.

STAGING

According to the sixth edition of the *AJCC Cancer Staging Manual*,[8] the pathologic staging is based on examination of the resected specimen. Although the extent of resection is not part of the TNM staging system, it is a prognostic factor of great significance. The TNM staging is described in **Table 1**.

Hilar Cholangiocarcinoma

Hilar CCA is an uncommon presentation of a rare disease; the only potentially curative approach is surgical resection. Given its incidence, clinical experience and management strategies have been limited to specific high-volume hepatobiliary centers. Broadly stated, goals of the surgical management are to perform a potentially curative resection or at least to palliate symptoms of obstructive jaundice. In the present day, however, biliary decompression for palliation is achieved more optimally by endoscopic or interventional radiologic procedures rather than by surgical bypass, especially considering that many unresectable malignancies are too proximal for effective surgical bypass.

The hepatic hilum is an anatomically complex area; historical clinical experience resulted in low R0 resection rates with significantly high perioperative morbidity and mortality.[9] An aggressive surgical approach inclusive of routine hepatectomy, caudate lobe resection, selective same-setting pancreatoduodenectomy (PD), and portal vein resection all have been used to achieve potentially more curative resections based on selected clinical evidence. These advances in procedural and technical factors combined with a greater understanding of the natural history of the disease over the past decade have been associated with a trend toward improved survival rates. The key prognostic factor remains the ability to achieve an R0 complete tumor resection.[10]

In the planning of surgical resection, patient selection is based on established criteria for resectability and is a key component for achieving an adequate R0 resection.[11,12] The core criteria for patient selection largely are predicated on the preoperative evaluation, which should asses the presence and extent of extrabiliary disease, inclusive of local or distant metastasis; demonstrate the presence or absence of local invasion; and provide a detailed view of biliary ductal anatomy to direct postresectional reconstruction when indicated. Multimodality noninvasive imaging techniques have been used in recent years to preoperatively stage patients who have CCA.[13]

Table 1			
Stage grouping of extrahepatic bile duct cancer			
Definition of TNM			
Primary tumor (T)			
TX Primary cannot be assessed			
T0 No evidence of primary tumor			
Tis Carcinoma in situ			
T1 Tumor confined to the bile duct histologically			
T2 Tumor invades beyond the wall of the bile duct			
T3 Tumor invades the liver, gallbladder, pancreas, or unilateral branches of the portal vein or hepatic artery			
T4 Tumor invades any of the following: main portal vein, common hepatic artery, or adjacent structures, such as colon, stomach, duodenum, or abdominal wall.			
Regional lymph nodes (N)			
NX Regional lymph nodes cannot be assessed			
N0 No regional lumph nodes metastasis			
N1 Regional lymph node metastasis			
Distant metastasis (M)			
MX Distant metastasis cannot be assessed			
M0 No distant metastasis			
M1 Distant metastasis			
Stage 0	Tis	N0	M0
Stage IA	T1	N0	M0
Stage IB	T2	N0	M0
Stage IIA	T3	N0	M0
Stage IIB	T1	N1	M0
	T2	N1	M0
	T3	N1	M0
Stage III	T4	Any N	M0
Stage IV	Any T	Any N	M1

Evolution of surgical treatment

Historical clinical experience with surgical management of hilar CCA was dismal by current standards given the reported high R1 and R2 resection rates. With the advent of improved surgical techniques, such as portal vein embolization and two-stage hepatectomy, and better understanding of biliary anatomy and the patterns of lymphatic drainage and regional nodal metastases, combined with the evolution of novel technologies for safe and rapid parenchymal liver division, hepatic and biliary resection overall has become safer and more commonplace. Specifically to CCA, there has been a reported higher frequency of major hepatectomy inclusive of caudate lobe resections for hilar CCA. With increased rates of major resections there has been a reported increase in achievement of negative resection margins.[11,14,15]

The Japanese were among the first to adopt the addition of caudate lobe resection in concert with hepatic and hilar resection, thus achieving an improved R0 resection rate. This maneuver is based in great part on the demonstration of variable drainage and vascular anatomic considerations of the caudate lobe, which preclude potentially curative resection when not resected. The North American and European centers subsequently adopted this approach, which paralleled the later inclusion of portal vein resection and reconstruction when indicated.

One of the largest reported series of resected hilar CCA has been published by Nishio and colleagues.[15] In their report, 301 patients were treated over a 27-year period. In this series, the evolution of the surgical procedure and management is well represented with 10.8% mortality in the first 20 years and 2.5% since 2000. These outcomes occurring as hepatectomy and lymphadenectomy with routine resection of the caudate lobe evolved into their routine surgical approach. Over the reported interval, an R0 resection was obtained in 233 patients with a reported median survival of 2.3 years and a 5-year survival rate of 27%. Patients who had positive lymph node metastasis did poorly (median survival 1.5 years) compared with patients who had negative lymph nodes. In this series, 97 patients required portal vein resection to obtain R0 resection; this subset had a poorer prognosis (median survival 1.4 years) compared with patients requiring no vascular resection (median 2.4 years) in whom an R0 was obtained. Even these patients did better, however, than patients who were not resectable.[15]

In North America the principal clinical experience is from the Memorial Sloan-Kettering Cancer Center. Jarnagin and colleagues[11] summarized the experience with 225 patients evaluated and 80 patients undergoing resection. Sixty-two of the patients underwent liver resection, 22 of the patients underwent caudate lobe resection, and 9 underwent portal vein resection. Median survival was 16 months for all patients, including resectable and unresectable patients. Median survival after R0 resection was 42 months compared with 21 months for patients who had an R1 resection and only 10 months for patients who do did not undergo resection at all. The perioperative morbidity was reported at 64% and the mortality rate was 10% with most morbidities and fatalities associated with infectious complications or hepatic insufficiency.

One of the most common reasons for the inability to obtain R0 resection is involvement of the portal vein. Historically, portal vein resection was uncommon and treated with great trepidation, which in modern day has shifted to an almost commonplace component of the operation, owing largely to the advent of improved techniques and more experience. Portal vein resection has increased the number of patients who are offered surgery for this disease; however, this component of the procedure has increased risk and resultant morbidity. Neuhaus and colleagues[16] reported a series of 80 patients, 23 of whom required portal vein resection. The perioperative mortality was 8% for the entire series whereas it was 17% for patients who had vascular resection. Multivariate analysis of portal vein resection patients demonstrated improved prognosis after excluding patients who had R1/2 resections and perioperative deaths. This analysis led the investigators to propose the "no touch" technique, thereby increasing the number of portal vein resections.

Hemming and colleagues[14] reported 60 resections for hilar CCA, including 26 cases that included resection and reconstruction of portal vein. In this series, the mortality rates were not higher for vascular resections and the median survival was no different compared with patients who did not undergo vascular resection. Similarly, Hidalgo and colleagues[17] reported 41 patients who had hilar CCA requiring resection, with 17 patients requiring portal vein resection. Overall, in these high-volume centers, the trend is notable for lesser morbidity and mortality with portal vein resections. It is feasible, however, that these are modest cohorts of the larger experience and the definitive role for portal vein resection remains in evolution.

A well-discussed controversy in the management of CCA has been the role of preoperative biliary drainage as most patients present with significantly elevated bilirubin secondary to obstruction. With the advent of contrast-enhanced CT scans and good magnetic resonance cholangiopancreatography (MRCP) imaging, the road map of the biliary system preoperatively can be obtained by these two studies. Previously, percutaneous transhepatic cholangiography (PTC) was used with diagnostic and therapeutic intent. With less invasive techniques providing adequate information for diagnosis and procedural planning, however, the need for diagnostic PTC has lessened.

The proposed advantages of preoperative biliary drainage are varied; they not only decrease bilirubin levels but also decrease the risk for cholangitis, improve nutritional status, improve liver function and hence the hepatic reserve, facilitate postresection liver regeneration and hypertrophy, and optimize renal function, to name a few. The inherent disadvantages of biliary drainage are infection, potential for tumor seeding, and the morbidity associated with the procedure. Several studies were performed in the mid-1980s in an effort to define the role of preoperative biliary drainage but failed to establish set criteria.[18–20]

Yet another modality of treatment for hilar CCA, which is controversial but gaining momentum in select centers, is liver transplantation. Meyer and colleagues[21] from the group at University of Cincinnati published their experience with 207 patients who had known unresectable CCA. The 1-, 2- and 5-year survival rates were reported as 72%, 48%, and 23%, respectively. Fifty-one percent of patients had recurrence of their tumors after transplantation and 84% of recurrences occurred within 2 years of transplantation; 47% of recurrences developed in the allograft and 30% in the lungs. Survival after recurrence rarely was longer than 1 year; similar results have been reported from other centers.[22–24]

These encouraging results led to the evolution of combined pancreaticoduodenectomy with liver transplantation, with the intent of achieving a potentially increased rate of complete tumor clearance (R0). Unfortunately, combined pancreaticoduodenectomy with liver transplant resulted in prohibitive increased mortality (60-day mortality rate, 15%) with only minimal increase in survival.[25,26]

Using a different approach with a similar intent, the Mayo Clinic (Rochester, Minnesota) group initiated the use of neoadjuvant chemoradiotherapy followed by liver transplantation in 1993 with Rea and colleagues[27] publishing the experience in 2005. In this series, patients who had T3/4 tumors and patients who had lymph node involvement (stage 3) had a poor prognosis. Also reported, however, was a series of 71 patients who had stage 1 or 2 CCA whose tumors were unresectable or arose in a background of primary sclerosing cholangitis (PSC). In this subset, protocol exclusion criteria were defined as advanced tumors (stage 3 or 4), tumors that extended below the cystic duct, and the presence of extrahepatic disease. Seventy-one patients were treated with neoadjuvant chemotherapy (5-fluorouracil followed by capecitabine), external beam radiotherapy (4500 cGy in 30 fractions), and percutaneous transhepatic brachytherapy (2000–3000 cGy). After neoadjuvant therapy, patients were restaged with laparotomy before transplantation. Overall, 38 (53%) patients underwent transplantation and the 1-, 3-, and 5-year survival rates were 92%, 82%, and 82%, respectively. It is notable that 16 of 38 explanted livers did not demonstrate any evidence of tumor and of these, only one half of the patients had a cancer diagnosis before treatment, which, as expected, has led to criticism of this study. Rosen and colleagues[28] recently updated this experience with 148 patients enrolled in a neoadjuvant protocol, 90 of whom have completed treatment. In this retrospective study over 14 years, of the 90 completed, 71 are still alive and 19 have died; however, only 8 of 19 deaths were from recurrent CCA.

Despite these exciting results, the neoadjuvant approach followed by liver transplantation is a difficult treatment modality to pursue on a large scale, given the already existing limitation in transplant organ availability.

Laparoscopic assessment

The role for laparoscopic assessment of extrabiliary disease in the treatment algorithm of hilar CCA has not been finalized. The literature supports that approximately 25% to 50% of affected patients are defined as unresectable by preoperative workup and an additional 30% to 50% further excluded by laparotomy.[11,14,29,30] As such it would be a general consensus that the majority of patients present with advanced unresectable disease.[11] Because the only potential procedures offered for these patients are palliative in nature, the argument is made that patients diagnosed with advanced stage by laparotomy undergo unnecessary laparotomy. In this era of radiologic PTC and endoscopic biliary drainage, as with other hepato-pancreato-biliary malignancies, only a few of these patients are expected to require a surgical bypass.[31]

Weber and colleagues[32] reported their experience for staging laparoscopy in the setting of hilar CCA and observed that 25% of the patients in the series could avoid an unnecessary laparotomy. Connor and colleagues[33] performed a combination of staging laparoscopy and intraoperative ultrasound (US) with a reported 42% decrease in unnecessary laparotomy for this disease. Weber and colleagues did not report a benefit for intraoperative US whereas the Connors and colleagues experience did.

Middle and Distal Cholangiocarcinoma

Patients who have extrahepatic CCA with a middle or distal site of origin usually present at a late stage of the disease, with 5-year survival less than 20%.[34] Definitive management of middle and distal CCA is surgical, with chemotherapy and radiotherapy having only a limited role. Potentially curative operation for distal CCA is reported to occur in 67% to 90% of resectable patients with an associated 5-year survival rate of 24% to 28%, which compares favorably with that reported for resection of hilar CCA.[5,35] The goal of surgical treatment is the complete resection of the tumor; however, the issue of optimal resection margins remains controversial.

Reported prognostic factors for distal extrahepatic CCA include surgical margin,[36] lymphatic invasion,[37] postoperative adjuvant chemotherapy,[36] and pathologic tumor differentiation grade.[5]

Identification of the tumor location and the extent of disease is a key factor for surgical planning. Preoperative radiologic evaluation includes US, CT, MRCP, endoscopic retrograde cholangiopancreatography, and PTC. US demonstrates the level of the biliary duct obstruction and provides information regarding tumor extension within the bile duct and the periductal tissues. Duplex US is useful for evaluating portal vein invasion. CT scan evaluates tumor involvement, vascular invasion, and liver atrophy. MRCP identifies the tumor, provides information about the patency of vascular structures, and evaluates for the presence of nodal or distant metastasis. Shi and colleagues[38] reported the accuracy of US, CT, MRCP in and detecting extrahepatic CCA as 81.25%, 87.29%, and 88.68%, respectively. Radiologic evaluation fails to clearly identify unresectable patients in approximately 60% of cases, which results in a large group of patients who have an intended curative resection having microscopic (R1) or macroscopic (R2) margins.[39]

Tissue diagnosis can be obtained preoperatively using endoscopic techniques. The choledochoscope-directed biopsy technique is reported to have greater sensitivity and specificity compared with the brush biopsies or biopsies obtained using the flexible clamshell (bioptome) forceps under fluoroscopic guidance.[40]

SURGICAL APPROACH
Limitation of Surgical Resection

Surgery with intent of complete resection is the only potentially curative treatment for CCA. Factors associated with unresectable hilar CCA have been reported and defined in multiple studies.[11,32] For middle/distal bile duct cancer, there is no consensus to clarify local extension factors associated with unresectable cases. Some studies reported combined portal vein resection[41] and hepatic artery resection[42] in an attempt to obtain a curative resection. Roder and colleagues[41] assessed the morbidity, mortality, and prognosis of PD in 31 patients in whom a tangential excision (n = 9) or a segmental resection (n = 22) of the portal vein or superior mesenteric vein was performed in an attempt to achieve complete tumor removal in patients who had peri-ampullary cancer. Despite no postoperative mortality, all patients who had pancreatic or bile duct carcinoma (n = 29) died within 16 months of the resection (median survival 8 months). In contrast, two patients who had cystadenocarcinoma and acinous cell carcinoma are alive with no evidence of recurrence at 23 and 54 months, respectively. The study concluded that portal vein resection does not prolong survival in patients undergoing partial PD for carcinoma of the pancreas or distal bile duct.

Kondo and colleagues[42] reported the feasibility and safety of arterioportal shunting as an alternative to arterial reconstruction after en bloc hepatic artery resection in 10 patients, including six patients who had bile duct carcinoma. An end-to-side arterio-portal reconstruction between the common hepatic or gastroduodenal artery and the portal trunk was performed in these cases. There was no operative mortality and postoperative complications included bile leakage in two patients and liver abscess in one. Routine angiography performed 1 month after surgery revealed shunt occlusion in three patients. Once the existence of hepatopedal arterial collaterals had been confirmed in the remaining patients, the shunt was occluded by coil emboliza-tion. Although the feasibility of the procedure was reported, its safety and its potential to increase the cure rate require further assessment in a larger series with a longer follow-up.

Metastatic disease to the liver, lung, peritoneum, and distant lymph nodes are considered stage 4 and exclude resection for hilar CCA and gallbladder cancer.[32] Altlernatively, there is no consensus to date on similarly limiting resection based on locoregional nodal involvement for distal CCA.

Surgical Modalities

For middle and lower CCA, complete surgical resection usually can be achieved by PD to assure negative margins and include local lymph nodes. If the cancer is localized, however, there is no evidence of lymph node metastasis, and negative margins can be intraoperatively assessed and achieved, a segmental bile duct resection (BDR) with Roux-en-Y reconstruction has been described. Jang and colleagues[43] reported no significant difference in 5-year survival between PD and BDR for T1 lesions with histo-logic findings of the papillary type or well-differentiated adenocarcinoma.

A more aggressive approach consisting of hepatopancreatoduodenectomy (HPD), which is en bloc hepatic resection with PD, may be indicated in CCA with longitudinal spread from the hepatic duct to the intrapancreatic duct. Nimura and colleagues[44] reported high mortality after HPD in 24 patients who had advanced gallbladder cancer or extrahepatic CCA. In this study, including nine patients who had CCA, 11 kinds of hepatic lobectomy or segmentectomy with PD were performed. The mortality rate was 35% with only 6% 5-year survival. In other studies, however, the mortality rate and the outcome after HPD were comparable to those with PD. In a retrospective comparative study, Yoshimi and colleagues[45] found that 30-day morality rate was 0% for 43 patients after PD and 13 patients after HPD for CCA; moreover, the long-term survival was not statistically different between the two groups. The same findings were supported by Kaneoaka and colleagues[46] who studied the outcome of 10 patients after HPD (five extended right and five extended left hepatectomies) for CCA with superficial spreading tumor or tumor with intramural or hepatoduodenal ligament invasion; the study reported 0% operative mortality and 64% 5-year survival after HPD.

In a few studies, total pancreatectomy (TP) was reported in the treatment of patients who had middle and lower segment CCA.[47,48] The procedure, although technically simpler than PD, carried a higher morbidity and mortality rate, without improvement in long-term survival.[47] Recent studies abandoned TP as a treatment modality. Studies reporting surgical management of extrahepatic middle and lower third CCA are reported in **Table 2**.

Hernandez and colleagues[49] studied 43 patients presenting with extrahepatic CCA, including eight patients who had middle segment CCA and 35 patients who had distal segment CCA. Patients who had mid tumors underwent BDR alone and patients who had distal tumors underwent PD. In this study, the overall survival was 21 months. Survival rate was not affected by tumor location or the margin status. Nodal status did not have an impact on survival when patients were stratified by margin status. The 30-day survival was 100% in the mid tumor and 91% in the distal tumor. There were no complications among patients undergoing BDR for mid tumors and postoperative morbidity in patients undergoing PD was 43%. This study suggested that microscopically positive margins after tumor resection may not represent a rapidly aggressive cancer with the investigators noting that CCAs are biologically indolent but relentless, given the observation that CCA-associated mortality is characteristically a slow progression of locoregional disease. As such, the presence of microscopic positive margins may not have an impact on overall survival. In this study, the use of adjuvant chemoradiation (5-fluorouracil with adjuvant radiotherapy) was not protocol driven, resulting in a minority of patients receiving adjuvant therapy. This concept is contradictory to other studies that have shown survival rates are different in patients who have micro- versus macroresidual tumors[50] and that 10- to 20-mm margins are required for eradication of invasive extrahepatic bile duct carcinoma.[51]

Shi and coworkers,[38] in a retrospective evaluation of surgical approach for extrahepatic CCA, showed that radical resection is the first choice for treatment. The tumor was located in the hilum in 80 patients, in the middle segment of the common bile duct in six patients, and in the inferior segment of the common bile duct in 39 patients. Ten patients had total common bile duct tumors. Radical resection was the treatment of choice for these patients, with a resection rate of 52.7% for patients who had hilar CCA, and a resection rate of 60.7% for patients who had middle and inferior CCA. Radical resection included variations of PD, BDR (with Roux-en-Y reconstruction), HPD, and liver resection, and a few patients (five) had liver transplant. Although the study did not dissect the survival for the group of patients who had hilar CCA and those who had mid or distal CCA, the overall survival for all patients at 1, 3, and 5 years was 46.9%, 37.3%, and 18.7%, respectively. The 1-, 3-, and 5-year survival rates in the radical resection group (74.9%, 55.7%, and 41.2%, respectively) were statistically better than those in the palliative resection group (42.8%, 26.7%, and 26.7%, respectively). The group of patients undergoing palliative drainage or nonoperation had the worst 1-, 3-, and 5-year survival rates of 23.3%, 6.67%, and 0%, which were statistically lower than the palliative surgery group. Multivariate analysis of outcome factors in these patients revealed that the histopathologic grade, TNM stage, and surgical modality were key factors. The surgical modality used was the prominent factor.

Woo and colleagues[52] reported, in a comparative study between distal CCA and ampullary cancer, that the 5-year survival of patients who had distal extrahepatic CCA after curative resection was 54%. Among the 91 patients who had distal extrahepatic CCA, 37 patients (41%) received adjuvant chemoradiotherapy and 35 patients (39%) experienced recurrence during the follow up. The most common patterns of recurrence were locoregional recurrence and liver metastasis. Tumor recurrence after radical resection invariably leads to death. According to univariate analysis the significant risk factors for distal extrahepatic CCA recurrence were abdominal pain, high CA 19-9 level, histologic grade, and lymph node involvement; multivariate analysis identified only lymph node involvement as significant.

The Role of Laparoscopic Surgery

To date, there is no study reporting the specific role of laparoscopy in the diagnosis, staging, or treatment of mid and distal CCA. Weber and colleagues[32] reported a role in staging laparoscopy for gallbladder cancer and hilar CCA. Although the yield from the laparoscopy was lower in the hilar CCA group than the gallbladder cancer group (25% and 48%, respectively), they suggested that all patients who have potentially resectable primary gallbladder cancer and patients who have T2/T3 hilar CCA should undergo staging laparoscopy before surgical exploration.

PROGNOSTIC FACTORS AFTER SURGICAL TREATMENT

Several studies reporting surgical experience in extrahepatic CCA have attempted to identify prognostic factors using multivariate analysis. Reported prognostic factors include presence of lymph node metastasis, surgical margins, tumor grading and morphology, and postoperative adjuvant therapy.

Nodal Involvement

The frequency of lymph node metastasis in distal CCA ranges from 30% to 68%.[5,36,37,53,54] Lymph node dissection in patients undergoing pylorus-preserving pancretoduodenectomy or conventional PD include nodes along the hepatic and celiac arteries, nodes in the hepatoduodenal and posterior pancreaticoduodenal nodes, and nodes on the right portion of the superior mesenteric artery; some series reported extensive nodal dissection to the para-aortic lymph nodes.[55] The presence of lymph node metastasis was found to be a negative prognostic factor in several studies.[5,36,37,54,55] The effect of positive lymph nodes on patient survival is reported on **Table 3**.

The number of involved lymph nodes has been reported to be a significant prognostic factor by univariate analysis.[36,56] In these series, patients who had up to two positive lymph nodes had a more favorable prognosis than patients who had three or more positive nodes (13% and 0% 5-year survival rates, respectively). Patients who had three or more lymph nodes frequently developed recurrence and distant metastasis to the liver, lung, and peritoneum.[36,56] Sasaki and colleagues[53] reported that patients who had distal CCA exhibiting nodal involvement had a significantly higher rate of liver metastasis than those who did not have nodal involvement. There is no report in the literature aborting a surgical resection based on the extent of lymph node disease.

Table 2
Studies reporting surgical treatment of middle and distal segment cholangiocarcinoma

Study (Publication Year)	Number of Patients	Number of Resected Patients	Curative Resection	Surgical Mortality	Median Survival (Months)	5-Year Survival(%)	Significant Prognostic Factors
Hernandez et al. (2008)[49]	43	43:35 PD, 8 BDR	R0 86% 75%	09%	21	—	Staging, adjuvant therapy
Murkami et al. (2007)[55]	43	43:35 PD, 8 BDR	R0 70%	0	26	44%	LN, SM
Ben-David et al. (2006)[60]	24	24	R0 16.7%	—	15.7	—	SM
Wakai et al. (2005)[57]	84	84:48 HBR, 19 PD, 9 BDR, HPD 8	R0 76%	3.6%	—	42%	LN, pM, Size and grade of tumor
Jang et al. (2005)[43]	282	151:103 PD, 25 BDR, 23 HBR	—	4.9% (all after PD)	—	32.5%	LN, histology, AJCC staging
Sakomoto et al. (2005)[85]	50	50:42 PD, 8 BDR	R0 74%	7%	38	26%	pT, BT
Park et al. (2004)[86]	59	59:48 PD, 11 BDR	R0 100%	0	45	47%	—
Yoshida et al. (2002)[36]	27	27 PD	R0 85%	4%	21	37%	LN, SM, AC
Sasaki et al. (2001)[53]	59	59:56 PD, 3 BDR	R0 85%	0	—	34%	—
Todorki et al. (2001)[61]	67	57:57 BDR, including 50 PD	R0 46%	5%	37	39%	Age, SM
Suzuki et al. (2000)[87]	99	99:79 PD, 20 BDR	R0 79%	3%	—	37%	—
Takao et al. (1999)[88]	64	64 PD	R0 66%	—	—	32%	Vascular invasion
Kayahara et al. (1999)[37]	50	50:43 PD, 7 BDR	R0 72%	2%	—	35%	LN, SM
Zerbi et al. (1998)[89]	27	27 PD	R0 96%	4%	22	13%	LI
Yeo et al. (1998)[59]	30	30 PD	R0 93%	—	22	27%	Tumor grade, SM, LN

Study							
Wade et al. (1997)[90]	34	34:30 PD, 4 BDR	—	11%	—	14%	—
Fong et al. (1996)[54]	104	45:39 PD, 6 BDR	R0 86%	4%	33	27%	LN
Nakeeb et al. (1996)[5]	73	73 PD	R0 90%	0	22	28%	LN, pG
Nagorney et al. (1993)[91]	39	22 PD	R0 56%	—	24	40%	—
Reding et al. (1991)[92]	172	84:51 PD, 31 BDR, 2 HBR	R0:46% middle, 50% distal	23% middle, 26% lower	13 middle, 34 lower	—	Location, TNM
Michelassi et al. (1989)[93]	40	36	R0 25%	10%	—	0%	Histology, SM
Tarazi et al. (1986)[94]	—	11 PD	—	0	—	17%	Histology
Lerut et al. (1984)[95]	5	5 PD	—	—	11	0%	—
Alexander et al. (1984)[96]	14	14	—	21%	16	18%	Tumor location, grading, complete resection
Herter et al. (1982)[47]	21	10:9 PD, 1 TP	—	—	55.3	33.3%	—
Tompkins et al. (1981)[35]	18	12	—	8%	18	28%	Tumor location
Nakase et al. (1977)[48]	309	161:157 PD, 4 TP	—	22%	17	5%	—
Warren et al. (1975)[97]	47	47 PD	R0 87.5%	17.4%	—	25%	LN

Abbreviations: HBR, hepatobiliary resection; LI, lymphatic invasion; LN, lymph node involvement; pT, pathologic staging of the tumor; pM, pathologic evidence of distant metastasis; SM, surgical margin.

Table 3
Studies evaluating the effect of lymph node involvement on patient survival after surgical resection of middle and distal cholangiocarcinoma

Study	Number of Patients	Lymph Node Positive 5-Year Survival	Lymph Node Positive 5-Year Survival
Murakami et al. (2007)[56]	43	58%	21%
Yoshida et al. (2002)[36]	27	60%	31%
Kayahara et al. (1999)[37]	50	65%	21%
Fong et al. (1996)[54]	45	54%	0%
Nakeeb et al. (1996)[5]	73	30%	10%

Surgical Margin

Surgical margin status has been reported to be a significant independent prognostic factor.[36,37,55,57] The beneficial effect of obtaining negative surgical margins is reported in **Table 4**.

Intraductal tumor spread for middle and lower CCA and the required margin length was evaluated in several studies. Shimada and colleagues[39] reported a mean intramural extension length of 16.8 mm. Yamaguchi and colleagues[58] reported a mean distance between the macroscopic tumor border estimated by cholangiography and the histologic tumor border was 6.1 mm proximally and 6.2 mm distally.

A retrospective pathologic study of 253 resected specimens of extrahepatic bile duct carcinoma[51] reported that the microscopic extension of invasive carcinoma beyond the macroscopically evident tumor mass was limited to 10 mm (75th percentile: 19.5 and 14.5 mm in proximal and distal directions, respectively; maximum 52 mm). Additional removal of any noninvasive component requires a 20-mm margin, however.

Tumor Grade and Histologic Findings

Tumor grading was found to be a significant prognostic factor in multivariable analysis in multiple studies. Yeo and colleagues[59] reported that the degree of tumor differentiation is a statistically significant prognostic factor after resection of CCA. Nakeeb and colleagues[5] reported a hazard ratio of 44% for poorly differentiated distal CCAs.

Table 4
Studies evaluating the effect of negative surgical margins on patient survival after surgical treatment of middle and distal segment cholangiocarcinoma

Study	Number of Patients	5-Year Survival (Negative Margin)	5-Year Survival (Positive Margin)
Murakami et al. (2007)[55]	43	60%	8%
Wakai et al.[a] (2005)[57]	84	46%	0% with invasive carcinoma 69% with carcinoma in situ
Yoshida et al. (2002)[36]	27	44%	0%
Kayahara et al. (1999)[37]	50	48%	0%

[a] Study of extrahepatic CCA include hilar and distal CCA.

PATTERNS OF FAILURE

Locoregional recurrence is the most common site of first failure after surgical treatment of mid and distal CCA. Ben-David and colleagues[60] reported that locoregional recurrence accounts for 60% of failure, followed by locoregional with distal and distal only in 20% of cases of each. The study suggested that surgery should be attempted only if surgical free margin can be obtained, although the use of postoperative radiotherapy or chemotherapy in patients who had positive resection margin could extend life. They suggested that patients who had borderline resectable tumors might benefit from neoadjuvant therapy. The importance of locoregional pattern of failure is consistent with Wakai and colleagues'[57] study reporting that among 11 patients who had positive ductal margins with carcinoma in situ, four died of tumor recurrence, two died from other causes, and five survived without disease. In all patients who died of the disease, the initial site of disease recurrence was local, suggesting that carcinoma in situ at ductal resection margins may be associated with local recurrence.

Alternatively, Hernandez and colleagues[49] suggested that most CCAs are biologically indolent and that the presence of positive margins may not have an impact on overall survival. The study reported survival of patients who had microscopically positive margins beyond 10 years.

Todoroki and colleagues[61] analyzed the predictors of metastasis after surgical resection of middle and lower third bile duct cancer. According to this study, all metastatic disease occurred in the liver and the only predicting factor was the presence of vascular invasion in the primary tumor. No significant correlation was found between the postoperative development of liver metastasis and lymphatic or perineural invasion.

PALLIATIVE MANAGEMENT

Biliary obstruction is a major problem and cause of morbidity and its palliation is a priority. The goal of a palliative therapy is relief of jaundice and related pruritis, prevention of cholangitis and hepatic dysfunction, and improvement of quality of life.[62] Biliary drainage can be achieved with equal efficiency by surgical biliary bypass, percutaneous drainage, or endoscopic drainage.[63] Smith and colleagues,[64] in a randomized trial of endoscopic stenting versus surgical bypass, found that the former offers significantly lower morbidity, mortality, and cost. For middle and lower segment CCA, metal stents provide longer patency and a more cost-effective measure for patients surviving at least 3 months.[65]

Another promising palliative modality is photodynamic therapy (PDT), which aims to reduce the tumor growth. Ortner and colleagues[66] in a randomized study reported a higher survival in patients managed with PDT than those managed with stents. The concomitant use of PDT and stenting showed promising results in hilar CCA. Witzigman and colleagues[67] reported that PDT plus stenting had similar survival for patients who had surgical R1 resection.

To date there is no study comparing the survival benefit of PDT with stenting to incomplete surgical resection in distal CCAs.

THE ROLE OF CHEMORADIOTHERAPY

Hejna and colleagues[68] in a meta-analysis study showed no benefit for patients who had CCA treated with 5-fluorouracil or mitomycin C alone or in combination with doxorubicin. New regimens, such as capecitabine and gemcitabine alone or combined with cisplatin, seem more effective.[69,70]

Pitt and colleagues[71] also showed in their prospective trial that adjuvant radiotherapy failed to show any survival or quality-of-life benefits in patients who had perihilar CCA. A relatively new radiotherapy approach using 3-D radiotherapy alone or in combination with chemotherapy as adjuvant treatment after surgical resection or as primary therapy has been reported for distal unresectable CCA.[68,72] Ben-David and colleagues,[60] in a series of 24 patients who had distal extrahepatic CCA, all receiving postoperative 3-D radiotherapy (54.0 Gy after R0 resection-54.9 Gy after R1 resection and 60.4 Gy after R2 resection), reported a median overall survival of 14.7 months. In this study there was no difference in outcome between R1 and R2 resection and 68% of recurrence was related to locoregional patterns of failure, suggesting that resection should be attempted only when an R0 resection is likely and that borderline resectable patients might benefit from neoadjuvant therapy. These findings remain controversial as other studies advocate a more aggressive surgical approach for distal CCA, reporting some benefit from R1 resection. Hernandez and colleagues[49] reported patients who had R1 resection receiving postoperative adjuvant therapy and surviving beyond 10 years; Jang and colleagues[43] also reported some patients who had R1 resection surviving after 5 years after chemoradiotherapy.

In the absence of a randomized controlled trial of postoperative adjuvant therapy versus R1 resection in patients who have locally advanced disease where complete resection cannot be obtained, it is difficult to define the optimal treatment algorithm in this group of patients. No study has assessed the feasibility and outcome of neoadjuvant therapy for unresectable distal CCA followed by a surgical resection.

THE ROLE OF PROPHYLACTIC SURGERY

Risk factors for development of CCA are age, PSC,[73] pancreatobiliary maljunction (PBM) with bile duct dilation,[74] chronic choledocholithiasis, biliary duct adenoma, biliary papillomatosis, Caroli's disease, choledochal cyst, smoking, parasitic infestation, and chronic typhoid carrier state. Most of the CCA, however, arise in the absence of any underlying risk factor.

Tashiro and colleagues[75] found that the incidence of biliary cancer is 10.6% (33% of these patients developed CCA) in patients who had PBM with bile duct dilatation. In patients who have PBM with bile duct dilatation prophylactic, excision of the gallbladder and the extrahepatic biliary duct should be considered.[76] For patients who have PBM without bile duct dilation, the need for prophylactic BDR is controversial.

Choledochal cyst predisposing to CCA is known, with adults more than 20 years old demonstrating the highest risk for developing CCA, with an incidence of up to 14%.[77-79] Prophylactic surgery is indicated in this group of patients who have excision of the entire dilated biliary tree and with reconstruction by Roux-en-Y hepaticojejunostomy.[77,78]

Patients who have PSC have a substantial predisposition to develop bile duct carcinoma. There still is no effective medical therapy that can halt the progression of the disease or prevent the development of CCA. The only effective treatment for advanced PSC is orthotopic liver transplantation (OLT), which, in the absence of CCA, has a 5-year survival of 89%. Patients who have CCA and who undergo OLT have a high risk for recurrence and a dramatically worsened survival. Therefore, the identification of patients who have a sufficient deterioration in liver function to warrant OLT before they develop CCA remains a central goal in the management of PSC.[80]

THE VALUE OF TUMOR MARKERS IN EARLY DETECTION OF CHOLANGIOCARCINOMA

Serologic tests for early detection of CCA have in general little value. Woo and colleagues[52] reported the value of elevated tumor markers in patients who have extrahepatic CCA. In their study of 91 patients who had distal CCA, 62% of patients had CA 19-9 levels greater than 37 U/mL and 10% of patients had carcinoembryonic antigen (CEA) levels greater than 5 ng/mL. Shi and colleagues also reported an elevated CA 19-9 in 72% of the patients who had extrahepatic cholangiocarcinoma.[38] Among different serum markers, including CEA and CA-125, the CA 19-9 was found (by the authors) the most useful, with a sensitivity and specificity of 67.5% and 86.8%, respectively; the specificity was found higher (96%) in patients who had peripheral CCAs using a CA 19-9 cutoff value greater than 100 kU/L. A CA 19-9 value greater than 600 kU/L was associated with nonresectable tumors.[81] As such, it has been suggested that serum CA 19-9 is of potential use the diagnosis of CCA, for deciding whether or not the tumor has been completely resected and for surveillance monitoring of the effect of treatment.[82,83] The low sensitivity of CA 19-9 and CEA is a limiting factor for the detection of CCA in patients who have PSC.[84]

REFERENCES

1. Pitt HA, Dooley WC, Yeo CJ, et al. Malignancies of the biliary tree. Curr Probl Surg 1995;32(1):1–90.
2. Khan SA, Taylor-Robinson SD, Toledano MB, et al. Changing international trends in mortality rates for liver, biliary and pancreatic tumours. J Hepatol 2002;37(6): 806–13.
3. Shaib YH, Davila JA, McGlynn K, et al. Rising incidence of intrahepatic cholangiocarcinoma in the United States: a true increase? J Hepatol 2004;40(3):472–7.
4. Kondo S, Takada T, Miyazaki M, et al. Guidelines for the management of biliary tract and ampullary carcinomas: surgical treatment. J Hepatobiliary Pancreat Surg 2008;15(1):41–54.
5. Nakeeb, A, Pitt, HA, Sohn, TA, et al. Cholangiocarcinoma. A spectrum of intrahepatic, perihilar, and distal tumors 1996 Ann Surg 224(4):463–73, [discussion 473–5].
6. Bismuth H, Corlette MB. Intrahepatic cholangioenteric anastomosis in carcinoma of the hilus of the liver. Surg Gynecol Obstet 1975;140(2):170–8.
7. Lim JH, Park CK. Pathology of cholangiocarcinoma. Abdom Imaging 2004;29(5): 540–7.
8. Greene FL, Page DL, Fleming ID, et al. AJCC cancer staging manual. 6th edition. New York: Springer; 2002.
9. Cameron JL, Pitt HA, Zinner MJ, et al. Management of proximal cholangiocarcinomas by surgical resection and radiotherapy. Am J Surg 1990;159(1):91–7 [discussion 97–8].
10. Saldinger PF, Blumgart LH. Resection of hilar cholangiocarcinoma—a European and United States experience. J Hepatobiliary Pancreat Surg 2000;7(2):111–4.
11. Jarnagin WR, Fong Y, DeMatteo RP, et al. Staging, resectability, and outcome in 225 patients with hilar cholangiocarcinoma. Ann Surg 2001;234(4):507–17 [discussion 517–9].
12. Vauthey JN, Blumgart LH. Recent advances in the management of cholangiocarcinomas. Semin Liver Dis 1994;14(2):109–14.
13. Chamberlain RS, Blumgart LH. Hilar cholangiocarcinoma: a review and commentary. Ann Surg Oncol 2000;7(1):55–66.
14. Hemming AW, Reed AI, Fujita S, et al. Surgical management of hilar cholangiocarcinoma. Ann Surg 2005;241(5):693–9 [discussion 699–702].
15. Nishio H, Nagino M, Nimura Y. Surgical management of hilar cholangiocarcinoma: the Nagoya experience. HPB (Oxford) 2005;7(4):259–62.

16. Neuhaus P, Jonas S, Bechstein WO, et al. Extended resections for hilar cholangiocarcinoma. Ann Surg 1999;230(6):808–18 [discussion 819].
17. Hidalgo E, Asthana S, Nishio H, et al. Surgery for hilar cholangiocarcinoma: the Leeds experience. Eur J Surg Oncol 2008;34(7):787–94.
18. Hatfield, AR, Tobias, R, Terblanche, J, et al. Preoperative external biliary drainage in obstructive jaundice. A prospective controlled clinical trial 1982 Lancet 2(8304):896–9.
19. McPherson GA, Benjamin IS, Hodgson HJ, et al. Pre-operative percutaneous transhepatic biliary drainage: the results of a controlled trial. Br J Surg 1984; 71(5):371–5.
20. Smith RC, Pooley M, George CR, et al. Preoperative percutaneous transhepatic internal drainage in obstructive jaundice: a randomized, controlled trial examining renal function. Surgery 1985;97(6):641–8.
21. Meyer CG, Penn I, James L. Liver transplantation for cholangiocarcinoma: results in 207 patients. Transplantation 2000;69(8):1633–7.
22. Shimoda M, Farmer DG, Colquhoun SD, et al. Liver transplantation for cholangiocellular carcinoma: analysis of a single-center experience and review of the literature. Liver Transpl 2001;7(12):1023–33.
23. Zheng SS, Huang DS, Wang WL, et al. Orthotopic liver transplantation in treatment of 77 patients with end-stage hepatic disease. Hepatobiliary Pancreat Dis Int 2002;1(1):8–13.
24. Robles R, Figueras J, Turrion VS, et al. Spanish experience in liver transplantation for hilar and peripheral cholangiocarcinoma. Ann Surg 2004;239(2):265–71.
25. Jonas S, Kling N, Guckelberger O, et al. Orthotopic liver transplantation after extended bile duct resection as treatment of hilar cholangiocarcinoma. First long-terms results. Transpl Int 1998;11(Suppl 1):S206–8.
26. Anthuber M, Schauer R, Jauch KW, et al. [Experiences with liver transplantation and liver transplantation combined with Whipple's operation in Klatskin tumor]. Langenbecks Arch Chir Suppl Kongressbd 1996;113:413–5.
27. Rea DJ, Heimbach JK, Rosen CB, et al. Liver transplantation with neoadjuvant chemoradiation is more effective than resection for hilar cholangiocarcinoma. Ann Surg 2005;242(3):451–8 [discussion 458–61].
28. Rosen CB, Heimbach JK, Gores GJ. Surgery for cholangiocarcinoma: the role of liver ransplantation. HPB (Oxford) 2008;10(3):186–9.
29. Mansfield SD, Barakat O, Charnley RM, et al. Management of hilar cholangiocarcinoma in the North of England: pathology, treatment, and outcome. World J Gastroenterol 2005;11(48):7625–30.
30. Launois B, Terblanche J, Lakehal M, et al. Proximal bile duct cancer. High resectability rate and 5-year survival. Ann Surg 1999;230(2):266–75.
31. Espat NJ, Brennan MF, Conlon KC. Patients with laparoscopically staged unresectable pancreatic adenocarcinoma do not require subsequent surgical biliary or gastric bypass. J Am Coll Surg 1999;188(6):649–55 [discussion 655–7].
32. Weber SM, DeMatteo RP, Fong Y, et al. Staging laparoscopy in patients with extrahepatic biliary carcinoma. Analysis of 100 patients. Ann Surg 2002;235(3): 392–9.
33. Connor S, Barron E, Wigmore SJ, et al. The utility of laparoscopic assessment in the preoperative staging of suspected hilar cholangiocarcinoma. J Gastrointest Surg 2005;9(4):476–80.
34. DeOliveira ML, Cunningham SC, Cameron JL, et al. Cholangiocarcinoma: thirty-one-year experience with 564 patients at a single institution. Ann Surg 2007; 245(5):755–62.

35. Tompkins RK, Thomas D, Wile A, et al. Prognostic factors in bile duct carcinoma: analysis of 96 cases. Ann Surg 1981;194(4):447–57.
36. Yoshida T, Matsumoto T, Sasaki A, et al. Prognostic factors after pancreatoduodenectomy with extended lymphadenectomy for distal bile duct cancer. Arch Surg 2002;137(1):69–73.
37. Kayahara M, Nagakawa T, Ohta T, et al. Role of nodal involvement and the periductal soft-tissue margin in middle and distal bile duct cancer. Ann Surg 1999; 229(1):76–83.
38. Shi QF, Liang TB, Qin YS, et al. Evaluation of surgical approach for extrahepatic cholangiocarcinoma. Hepatobiliary Pancreat Dis Int 2007;6(6):622–6.
39. Shimada H, Nimoto S, Nakagawara G, et al. [Infiltration of bile duct carcinoma along the wall]. Nippon Geka Gakkai Zasshi 1985;86(2):179–86.
40. Savader SJ, Prescott CA, Lund GB, et al. Intraductal biliary biopsy: comparison of three techniques. J Vasc Interv Radiol 1996;7(5):743–50.
41. Roder JD, Stein HJ, Siewert JR. Carcinoma of the periampullary region: who benefits from portal vein resection? Am J Surg 1996;171(1):170–4 [discussion 174–5].
42. Kondo S, Hirano S, Ambo Y, et al. Arterioportal shunting as an alternative to microvascular reconstruction after hepatic artery resection. Br J Surg 2004; 91(2):248–51.
43. Jang JY, Kim SW, Park DJ, et al. Actual long-term outcome of extrahepatic bile duct cancer after surgical resection. Ann Surg 2005;241(1):77–84.
44. Nimura Y, Hayakawa N, Kamiya J, et al. Hepatopancreatoduodenectomy for advanced carcinoma of the biliary tract. Hepatogastroenterology 1991;38(2): 170–5.
45. Yoshimi F, Asato Y, Amemiya R, et al. Comparison between pancreatoduodenectomy and hepatopancreatoduodenectomy for bile duct cancer. Hepatogastroenterology 2001;48(40):994–8.
46. Kaneoka Y, Yamaguchi A, Isogai M. Hepatopancreatoduodenectomy: its suitability for bile duct cancer versus gallbladder cancer. J Hepatobiliary Pancreat Surg 2007;14(2):142–8.
47. Herter FP, Cooperman AM, Ahlborn TN, et al. Surgical experience with pancreatic and periampullary cancer. Ann Surg 1982;195(3):274–81.
48. Nakase A, Matsumoto Y, Uchida K, et al. Surgical treatment of cancer of the pancreas and the periampullary region: cumulative results in 57 institutions in Japan. Ann Surg 1977;185(1):52–7.
49. Hernandez J, Cowgill SM, Al-Saadi S, et al. An aggressive approach to extrahepatic cholangiocarcinomas is warranted: margin status does not impact survival after resection. Ann Surg Oncol 2008;15(3):807–14.
50. Sasaki R, Takeda Y, Funato O, et al. Significance of ductal margin status in patients undergoing surgical resection for extrahepatic cholangiocarcinoma. World J Surg 2007;31(9):1788–96.
51. Ebata T, Watanabe H, Ajioka Y, et al. Pathological appraisal of lines of resection for bile duct carcinoma. Br J Surg 2002;89(10):1260–7.
52. Woo SM, Ryu JK, Lee SH, et al. Recurrence and prognostic factors of ampullary carcinoma after radical resection: comparison with distal extrahepatic cholangiocarcinoma. Ann Surg Oncol 2007;14(11):3195–201.
53. Sasaki R, Takahashi M, Funato O, et al. Prognostic significance of lymph node involvement in middle and distal bile duct cancer. Surgery 2001;129(6): 677–83.
54. Fong Y, Blumgart LH, Lin E, et al. Outcome of treatment for distal bile duct cancer. Br J Surg 1996;83(12):1712–5.

55. Murakami Y, Uemura K, Hayashidani Y, et al. Prognostic significance of lymph node metastasis and surgical margin status for distal cholangiocarcinoma. J Surg Oncol 2007;95(3):207–12.

56. Murakami Y, Uemura K, Hayashidani Y, et al. Pancreatoduodenectomy for distal cholangiocarcinoma: prognostic impact of lymph node metastasis. World J Surg 2007;31(2):337–42 [discussion 343–4].

57. Wakai T, Shirai Y, Moroda T, et al. Impact of ductal resection margin status on long-term survival in patients undergoing resection for extrahepatic cholangiocarcinoma. Cancer 2005;103(6):1210–6.

58. Yamaguchi K, Chijiiwa K, Saiki S, et al. Carcinoma of the extrahepatic bile duct: mode of spread and its prognostic implications. Hepatogastroenterology 1997; 44(17):1256–61.

59. Yeo CJ, Sohn TA, Cameron JL, et al. Analysis of 5-year survivors. Ann Surg 1998; 227(6):821–31.

60. Ben-David MA, Griffith KA, Abu-Isa E, et al. External-beam radiotherapy for localized extrahepatic cholangiocarcinoma. Int J Radiat Oncol Biol Phys 2006;66(3):772–9.

61. Todoroki T, Kawamoto T, Koike N, et al. Treatment strategy for patients with middle and lower third bile duct cancer. Br J Surg 2001;88(3):364–70.

62. Demols A, Marechal R, Deviere J, et al. The multidisciplinary management of gastrointestinal cancer. Biliary tract cancers: from pathogenesis to endoscopic treatment. Best Pract Res Clin Gastroenterol 2007;21(6):1015–29.

63. Abu-Hamda EM, Baron TH. Endoscopic management of cholangiocarcinoma. Semin Liver Dis 2004;24(2):165–75.

64. Smith AC, Dowsett JF, Russell RC, et al. Randomised trial of endoscopic stenting versus surgical bypass in malignant low bileduct obstruction. Lancet 1994; 344(8938):1655–60.

65. Kaassis M, Boyer J, Dumas R, et al. Plastic or metal stents for malignant stricture of the common bile duct? Results of a randomized prospective study. Gastroint-est Endosc 2003;57(2):178–82.

66. Ortner ME, Caca K, Berr F, et al. Successful photodynamic therapy for nonresectable cholangiocarcinoma: a randomized prospective study. Gastroenterology 2003;125(5):1355–63.

67. Witzigmann H, Berr F, Ringel U, et al. Surgical and palliative management and outcome in 184 patients with hilar cholangiocarcinoma: palliative photodynamic therapy plus stenting is comparable to r1/r2 resection. Ann Surg 2006;244(2): 230–9.

68. Hejna M, Pruckmayer M, Raderer M. The role of chemotherapy and radiation in the management of biliary cancer: a review of the literature. Eur J Cancer 1998;34(7):977–86.

69. Malik IA, Aziz Z, Zaidi SH, et al. Gemcitabine and Cisplatin is a highly effective combination chemotherapy in patients with advanced cancer of the gallbladder. Am J Clin Oncol 2003;26(2):174–7.

70. Patt YZ, Hassan MM, Aguayo A, et al. Oral capecitabine for the treatment of hepatocellular carcinoma, cholangiocarcinoma, and gallbladder carcinoma. Cancer 2004;101(3):578–86.

71. Pitt HA, Nakeeb A, Abrams RA, et al. Perihilar cholangiocarcinoma. Postoperative radiotherapy does not improve survival. Ann Surg 1995;221(6):788–97 [discussion 797–8].

72. Foo ML, Gunderson LL, Bender CE, et al. External radiation therapy and trans-catheter iridium in the treatment of extrahepatic bile duct carcinoma. Int J Radiat Oncol Biol Phys 1997;39(4):929–35.

73. Rosen CB, Nagorney DM. Cholangiocarcinoma complicating primary sclerosing cholangitis. Semin Liver Dis 1991;11(1):26–30.
74. Matsumoto Y, Fujii H, Itakura J, et al. Pancreaticobiliary maljunction: pathophysiological and clinical aspects and the impact on biliary carcinogenesis. Langenbecks Arch Surg 2003;388(2):122–31.
75. Tashiro S, Imaizumi T, Ohkawa H, et al. Pancreaticobiliary maljunction: retrospective and nationwide survey in Japan. J Hepatobiliary Pancreat Surg 2003;10(5):345–51.
76. Miyazaki M, Takada T, Miyakawa S, et al. Risk factors for biliary tract and ampullary carcinomas and prophylactic surgery for these factors. J Hepatobiliary Pancreat Surg 2008;15(1):15–24.
77. Jan YY, Chen HM, Chen MF. Malignancy in choledochal cysts. Hepatogastroenterology 2002;49(43):100–3.
78. Bismuth H, Krissat J. Choledochal cystic malignancies. Ann Oncol 1999;4(10 Suppl):94–8.
79. Voyles CR, Smadja C, Shands WC, et al. Carcinoma in choledochal cysts. Age-related incidence. Arch Surg 1983;118(8):986–8.
80. Harrison PM. Prevention of bile duct cancer in primary sclerosing cholangitis. Ann Oncol 1999;10(suppl 4):208–11.
81. John AR, Haghighi KS, Taniere P, et al. Is a raised CA 19-9 level diagnostic for a cholangiocarcinoma in patients with no history of sclerosing cholangitis? Dig Surg 2006;23(5–6):319–24.
82. Qin XL, Wang ZR, Shi JS, et al. Utility of serum CA19-9 in diagnosis of cholangiocarcinoma: in comparison with CEA. World J Gastroenterol 2004;10(3):427–32.
83. Patel AH, Harnois DM, Klee GG, et al. The utility of CA 19-9 in the diagnoses of cholangiocarcinoma in patients without primary sclerosing cholangitis. Am J Gastroenterol 2000;95(1):204–7.
84. Bjornsson E, Kilander A, Olsson R. CA 19-9 and CEA are unreliable markers for cholangiocarcinoma in patients with primary sclerosing cholangitis. Liver 1999;19(6):501–8.
85. Sakamoto Y, Kosuge T, Shimada K, et al. Prognostic factors of surgical resection in middle and distal bile duct cancer: an analysis of 55 patients concerning the significance of ductal and radial margins. Surgery 2005;137(4):396–402.
86. Park SW, Park YS, Chung JB, et al. Patterns and relevant factors of tumor recurrence for extrahepatic bile duct carcinoma after radical resection. Hepatogastroenterology 2004;51(60):1612–8.
87. Suzuki M, Unno M, Oikawa M, et al. Surgical treatment and postoperative outcomes for middle and lower bile duct carcinoma in Japan—experience of a single institute. Hepatogastroenterology 2000;47(33):650–7.
88. Takao S, Shinchi H, Uchikura K, et al. Liver metastases after curative resection in patients with distal bile duct cancer. Br J Surg 1999;86(3):327–31.
89. Zerbi A, Balzano G, Leone BE, et al. Clinical presentation, diagnosis and survival of resected distal bile duct cancer. Dig Surg 1998;15(5):410–6.
90. Wade TP, Prasad CN, Virgo KS, et al. Experience with distal bile duct cancers in U.S. Veterans Affairs hospitals: 1987–1991. J Surg Oncol 1997;64(3):242–5.
91. Nagorney DM, Donohue JH, Farnell MB, et al. Outcomes after curative resections of cholangiocarcinoma. Arch Surg 1993;128(8):871–7 [discussion 877–9].
92. Reding R, Buard JL, Lebeau G, et al. Surgical management of 552 carcinomas of the extrahepatic bile ducts (gallbladder and periampullary tumors excluded). Results of the French surgical association survey. Ann Surg 1991;213(3):236–41.

93. Michelassi F, Erroi F, Dawson PJ, et al. Experience with 647 consecutive tumors of the duodenum, ampulla, head of the pancreas, and distal common bile duct. Ann Surg 1989;210(4):544–54 [discussion 554–6].
94. Tarazi RY, Hermann RE, Vogt DP, et al. Results of surgical treatment of periampullary tumors: a thirty-five-year experience. Surgery 1986;100(4):716–23.
95. Lerut JP, Gianello PR, Otte JB, et al. Pancreaticoduodenal resection. Surgical experience and evaluation of risk factors in 103 patients. Ann Surg 1984; 199(4):432–7.
96. Alexander, F, Rossi, RL, O'Bryan, M, et al. Biliary carcinoma. A review of 109 cases 1984 Am J Surg 147(4): 503–9.
97. Warren KW, Choe DS, Plaza J, et al. Results of radical resection for periampullary cancer. Ann Surg 1975;181(5):534–40.

Management and Extent of Resection for Intrahepatic Cholangiocarcinoma

Darren R. Carpizo, MD, PhD[a], Michael D'Angelica, MD[b,c],*

KEYWORDS

- Intrahepatic cholangiocarcinoma • Resection
- Biliary cancer • Liver cancer

Cholangiocarcinomas are malignant neoplasms that arise from biliary epithelium anywhere along the biliary tract. They can be generally classified by anatomic location into intrahepatic (10%) and extrahepatic (hilar cholangiocarcinoma [HC] 50%–60%, distal bile duct 20%–30%). Intrahepatic cholangiocarcinoma (ICC) is the second most common primary liver malignancy behind hepatocellular carcinoma.[1] The etiology of ICC is poorly understood but several diseases that are associated with cholangiocarcinoma are linked by a common pathologic condition, chronic biliary inflammation. These include primary biliary cirrhosis; primary sclerosing cholangitis (PSC); chronic hepatolithiasis; choledochal cyst disease; hepatitis C viral infection; and parasitic biliary infestation (*Clonorchis sinensis* and *Opisthorchis viverrini*).

ICC remains a poorly understood cancer in part because it is a relatively rare tumor, particularly in the United States, where its incidence is approximately 0.67 per 100,000. There have been several reports documenting a significant increase in the incidence and mortality of ICC not only in the United States, but also in such countries as Japan and the United Kingdom.[2–4] When the incidence of ICC in the United States was examined using the Surveillance, Epidemiology and End Results (SEER) database from 1973 to 1997, it had increased by 9.1% over this time period (**Fig. 1**). This is a significant increase given that the incremental percent change for all digestive tract cancers combined during the same period was −0.32%.[2]

The factors responsible for the rising incidence in the United States are unclear. There has been no significant change in the incidence of risk factors associated

[a] Division of Surgery, UMDNJ-Robert Wood Johnson Medical School, The Cancer Institute of New Jersey, 195 Little Albany Street, Room 3040, New Brunswick, NJ 08901, USA
[b] Department of Surgery, Memorial Sloan-Kettering Cancer Center, 1275 York Avenue, NY 10021, USA
[c] Weill Medical College of Cornell University, New York, NY, USA
* Corresponding author. Department of Surgery, Memorial Sloan-Kettering Cancer Center, Weill Medical College of Cornell University, 1275 York Avenue, NY 10021, USA.
E-mail address: dangelim@mskcc.org (M. D'Angelica).

Surg Oncol Clin N Am 18 (2009) 289–305
doi:10.1016/j.soc.2008.12.010
1055-3207/08/$ – see front matter © 2009 Elsevier Inc. All rights reserved.

surgonc.theclinics.com

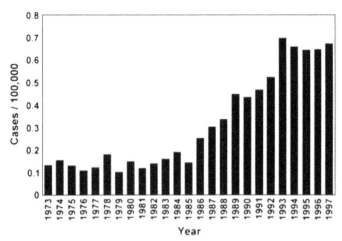

Year

Fig. 1. Age-adjusted (1970 United States standard) incidence rates of primary intrahepatic cholangiocarcinoma, 1973 to 1997. (*From* Patel T. Increasing incidence and mortality of primary intrahepatic cholangiocarcinoma in the United States. Hepatology 2001;33: 1353–72; with permission.)

with ICC. Recently, a high incidence of ICC has been reported in patients with cirrhosis related to hepatitis C in Japan.[5,6] This might be one explanation for the rise in the United States given the increasing numbers of patients with documented hepatitis C. Another explanation could be related to better recognition and diagnosis of ICC. In the past, patients with adenocarcinoma in the liver with no primary tumor were often referred to as "metastatic adenocarcinoma of unknown primary."

The most effective treatment for ICC is complete resection because systemic chemotherapy for this disease is ineffective. Unfortunately, this is possible in the minority of patients. Most patients present with unresectable disease either because of locally advanced or distant spread. Another problem in the United States is that many potentially resectable patients with localized disease may not be undergoing complete resection. In a study of the SEER database between 1988 and 2003, Tan and colleagues[7] identified 558 patients with ICC from a total of 6067 cases of cholangiocarcinoma. From this number they identified 248 cases of localized disease and found that only 37% underwent cancer-directed surgery. Cancer-directed surgery was broadly defined as any surgical intervention that has therapeutic intent. This could range from complete versus partial resection to ablative therapies. With the lack of surgical detail or documentation of reasons why cancer-directed surgery was not offered to specific patients it is difficult to make definitive conclusions from these data. Nonetheless, there is a strong suggestion that many patients with potentially curable disease may not be having surgery offered to them. This emphasizes the need for a better understanding of a disease whose incidence is rapidly rising.

This article reviews the literature pertinent to the surgical management of ICC. Issues pertaining to clinical presentation, preoperative work-up, extent of resection, and prognostic factors associated with outcome are discussed. Also commented on are treatment options in the unresectable patient.

PREOPERATIVE EVALUATION
Clinical Presentation, Work-up, and Imaging

Unlike extrahepatic biliary cancers that usually present with jaundice, ICC when symptomatic usually presents with right upper quadrant abdominal pain, weight loss or night sweats, and a liver mass on imaging. It is becoming more common that ICC presents as an incidental liver mass on imaging performed for other reasons. The most common presentation to a surgeon is that of a patient with a liver mass that has been biopsied elsewhere and found to be adenocarcinoma.

Given that most malignant liver masses in the United Stares are metastatic, a careful search for a primary tumor must be performed. This includes contrast-enhanced imaging of the chest, abdomen, and pelvis to rule out, among others, lung, pancreas, and gynecologic and urologic tumors. A colonoscopy and upper endoscopy should be performed to rule out an intraluminal gastrointestinal malignancy. Women should have a mammogram and routine gynecologic screening. Risk factors for primary hepatic malignancy should be assessed, in particular viral hepatitis, biliary disorders, alcohol abuse, and cirrhosis. Tumor markers, such as carcinoembryonic antigen, CA19-9, and alpha fetoprotein, are typically drawn. Careful pathologic review with an experienced pathologist is helpful to try to elucidate the nature of the malignancy. If a biopsy has not been performed and the work-up shows a malignant-appearing mass in the liver with no primary tumor, biopsy is not advocated because of potential complications and the risk of a false-negative finding.

Work-up with standard cross-sectional imaging includes multidetector, contrast-enhanced helical CT or MRI and MR cholangiopancreatography. Typical findings include a malignant-appearing irregular, heterogenous mass with peripheral biliary dilatation. Typical features found on CT include a rim-like contrast enhancement at the tumor periphery with areas of delayed contrast enhancement within the tumor. In addition, these tumors tend to be invasive of the hepatic and portal venous vasculature and cause peripheral biliary dilatation.[8]

On MRI, ICC appear hypointense relative to normal liver on T1-weighted images and relatively heterogenous on T2-weighted images.[9] Maetani and colleagues[10] studied 50 patients with ICC and correlated their MRI features to their histopathology. They found in 27 of 50 cases that ICC exhibited central areas of lower signal intensity compared with the tumoral edge on T2-weighted images. These areas correlated with fibrosis on pathology. This finding on MRI was just as common in metastatic colorectal tumors (16 of 34) but much less frequent in other hepatic tumors (26 of 234). The presence of intrahepatic biliary dilatation was observed in 27 of 50 patients with ICC, whereas it was seen in only 1 of 34 cases of metastatic colorectal cancer. ICC can look very similar to metastatic colorectal cancer on MRI and can be distinguished by the presence of intrahepatic biliary dilatation.

Serum Tumor Markers

Serum tumor markers typically evaluated include CA19-9, carcinoembryonic antigen, and CA-125. Of the three, CA19-9 is perhaps the most useful particularly in patients with PSC. When the value is greater than 100 U/mL, the sensitivity and specificity are 89% and 86%, whereas in patients without PSC, the sensitivity falls to 53%.[11] Overall, the role of tumor markers for ICC is minimally studied and there is very little information on its diagnostic accuracy and prognostic importance. Perhaps the most useful role is to measure levels before and after treatment to help assess efficacy and to screen for recurrence after normalization.

Positron Emission Tomography

The role of positron emission tomography (PET) and PET-CT in the management of patients with cholangiocarcinoma and specifically ICC remains poorly defined. Studies that have examined this issue are small in number and contain relatively few patients with ICC, usually mixed with other biliary cancers. Nonetheless, there is a suggestion that PET may enhance the detection of distant metastases in patients with ICC. Kim and colleagues[12] studied PET in 21 patients with biliary cancer (10 HC, 11 ICC) and compared it with conventional imaging with CT or MRI for the detection of the primary tumor, regional lymph node, and distant metastases. They found that PET tracer uptake was higher in ICC than for HC (mean SUV max 9.3 for ICC versus 4.4 for HC; $P<.05$) and was not beneficial in detecting regional lymph node metastases. PET did, however, identify 4 of 21 patients with occult distant metastases not seen on CT or MRI. All four of these patients had ICC.

The combination of CT and PET in a single examination has enhanced its accuracy in staging a number of solid organ cancers including lung, pancreas, and colorectal cancers.[13] Recently, PET-CT was compared with conventional contrast-enhanced CT in 61 patients with biliary cancers (gallbladder 14, ICC 14, HC 33).[13] The results were similar in that PET-CT was highly sensitive for detecting the primary tumor in ICC but this was no better than conventional CT (sensitivity 93% PET-CT versus 78% CT; $P = .59$). PET-CT was no better for the detection of regional lymph nodes for the entire cohort (sensitivity 12% PET-CT versus 24% CT; $P = .66$). A total of 12 (20%) of 61 patients, however, were found to have distant metastases and PET-CT detected all 12, whereas CT only detected 3 (sensitivity 100% PET-CT versus 25% CT; $P = .001$) (**Fig. 2**). Overall, in this study, PET-CT changed the management in 8 (17%) of 48 patients. The experience with PET or PET-CT and ICC remains too immature to recommend its inclusion as part of the standard work-up in a patient with ICC. Nonetheless, it seems that its benefit, if any, is in the identification of distant disease.

SURGICAL MANAGEMENT
Staging Laparoscopy

Despite the improvements in staging that have come from modern imaging, there still is a substantial number of patients with occult metastatic disease that manifest as

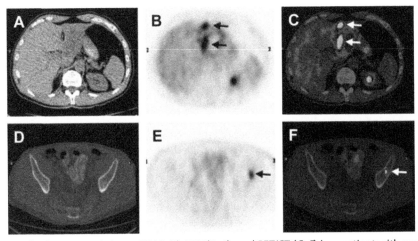

Fig. 2. The figure panel shows CT (*A, D*), PET (*B, E*), and PET/CT (*C, F*) in a patient with metastatic intrahepatic cholangiocarcinoma. A specific FDG accumulation in the primary tumor (*arrow*) in the left liver (*B, C*) and in a distant metastases in the left iliac bone (*E, F*) was detected. (*From* Petrowsky H, Wildbrett P, Husarik DB, et al. Impact of integrated positron emission tomography and computed tomography on staging and management of gallbladder cancer and cholangiocarcinoma. J Hepatol 2006;45:43–5013; with permission.)

either peritoneal or intrahepatic metastases found at operation. For this reason, staging laparoscopy has been advocated. Few studies have addressed the role of staging laparoscopy for ICC. Goere and colleagues[14] studied the yield of diagnostic laparoscopy in 39 patients with biliary cancer who were believed to be potentially resectable by preoperative imaging. Among the 11 patients in this study with ICC, 4 were found to be unresectable at laparoscopy for a yield of 36%. Weber and colleagues[15] reported a series of 53 patients with ICC, 22 of whom underwent diagnostic laparoscopy. They found six patients (27%) to be unresectable either because of peritoneal metastases (four) or additional intrahepatic tumors (two). Despite the small number of studies on diagnostic laparoscopy for ICC, the available data do indicate a sufficient yield that justifies its routine use.

Extent of Hepatic Resection

Because the most effective treatment for ICC is surgical resection, patients need to be examined for their overall fitness to undergo major hepatectomy. Particular attention should be made to medical comorbidities, presence of chronic liver disease, or portal hypertension. The goals of surgery should be complete surgical removal of the tumor with negative margins while leaving an adequate liver remnant volume. Because ICC is often asymptomatic, tumors can be quite large at diagnosis and technically challenging to resect. This may require an extended resection to involve nearby structures, such as the extrahepatic biliary tree, vascular structures, and the diaphragm or bowel.

Lang and colleagues[16] compared the operative findings and outcomes of 41 patients with ICC with 61 patients with hepatocellular carcinoma. All patients in this study underwent an R0 resection in a noncirrhotic liver and had no adjuvant therapy. They found the 5-year overall survival between the two groups to be approximately the same (44% for ICC, 40% for hepatocellular carcinoma; $P = .38$). When comparing the operative data, they found that the ICC patients required a more extensive liver resection (>32 hemihepatectomy, <9 hemihepatectomy) versus the hepatocellular carcinoma group (>34 hemihepatectomy, <27 hemihepatectomy; $P = .036$).

Although these tumors may require more extensive resections, it is unclear as to the importance of a negative margin. This issue was recently highlighted in a single institution series that reported results with 50 patients who all underwent surgical exploration for locally advanced ICC (tumors involving more than four liver segments requiring an extended hepatectomy).[16] Resection was performed in 27 (54%) of 50 cases. In 16 patients, the following additional 29 procedures were performed: resection of the hilar bifurcation (N = 12); diaphragm excision (N = 5); hepatic artery resection and reconstruction (N = 1); and resection and reinsertion of the left hepatic vein (N = 1). The 30-day mortality was 6% (3 of 27) and the morbidity was 52%. The median tumor diameter was 10 cm and an R0 resection was achieved in 16 patients, whereas 11 had an R1 resection.

With a median follow-up of 28 months, 13 of the 16 R0 patients are alive with a 1- and 3-year survival rate of 94% and 82%, respectively. In contrast, after R1 resection 8 of 11 patients died within 1 year. The authors concluded that an aggressive surgical approach including resection of vascular and biliary structures is justified if an R0 resection can be achieved. It must be noted that many of these patients had extensive vascular invasion, nodal metastases, and multifocal tumors and a multivariate analysis of factors associated with outcome was not performed. Definitive conclusions about margins that apply to resectable patients cannot be made.

Many other series have found that on multivariate analysis margin status is not associated with outcome (see later). This is likely because tumor-related factors, such as multifocality, vascular invasion, and nodal metastases, overwhelm outcome as poor prognostic factors. In general, a complete gross resection is advocated and, although a negative margin should be strived for it is probably not the most important predictor of outcome. Extensive resections as described previously are justified but should be performed in a center where such procedures are performed on a regular basis.

Portal Lymph Node Dissection

Several studies on ICC have identified portal lymph node metastases as a poor prognostic factor.[17–20] Whether or not a routine portal lymphadenectomy should be performed remains a controversial topic in the surgical management of ICC. The recommendations from various centers vary from routine portal lymphadenectomy to selective lymph node sampling to none at all. The arguments to perform lymphadenectomy are for staging purposes and to decrease regional nodal recurrence. There are very little data to support a therapeutic benefit to lymphadenectomy. Weber and colleagues[15] reported a small number of recurrences in the hilar nodes (3 of 20 recurrences) among 53 patients undergoing resection for ICC. They suggested that these recurrences may have been prevented by portal lymphadenectomy.

Shimada and colleagues[20] in a retrospective analysis of 49 patients undergoing resection for ICC compared recurrence patterns and outcomes of 41 patients who had portal lymphadenectomy with 8 patients who did not. They found 24 of 41 patients with portal lymph node metastases in the lymphadenectomy group. Twenty-three patients recurred and none had portal lymph node recurrences and the overall survival between the two groups was similar. They concluded that lymph node dissection was of no survival benefit and should not routinely be performed.

The authors have adopted a selective approach to portal lymphadenectomy because they have found that in the absence of any suspicion of portal node involvement on imaging (PET or CT-MRI) or intraoperative assessment, the incidence of portal lymph node involvement is too low to warrant routine lymphadenectomy.[21] This conclusion was based on a study of 100 patients with primary and secondary hepatic malignancies undergoing routine portal lymphadenectomy, 8 of whom had ICC.

Liver Transplantation

During the 1990s there was considerable enthusiasm for liver transplantation for primary liver cancers including cholangiocarcinoma. Although transplantation for hepatocellular carcinoma has become accepted as an effective treatment modality for patients with limited volume disease, the results with ICC have been poor causing many to consider transplantation a contraindication in ICC.[22,23]

Some studies have found encouraging long-term survival in patients with incidentally discovered cholangiocarcinomas in the explanted livers of patients with PSC.[24,25] This has suggested that survival after transplantation for ICC is better when the tumor is incidentally found or of an early stage. This issue was recently investigated by a Canadian group that reported the outcomes of 10 patients undergoing liver transplant and found incidentally to have discovered cholangiocarcinoma.[26] These patients accounted for 0.3% of all liver transplant patients and 3% of all patients with PSC undergoing transplantation among multiple centers. They found the 3-year overall survival to be 30%, with a median survival of 30 months. They concluded that patients with incidentally discovered cholangiocarcinoma had roughly the same outcomes as those historically who had undergone transplantation for clinically evident cholangiocarcinoma. These data further raise concerns about the role of transplantation for ICC even for the earliest stage tumors.

Recently, a group from the Mayo Clinic reported encouraging outcomes in patients with HC treated with neoadjuvant chemoradiation followed by liver transplantation.[27] These patients had unresectable HC or HC in the setting of PSC with no extrahepatic or lymph node metastases as determined by laparotomy. They enrolled 71 and transplanted 38 patients. The 3- and 5-year survival for this group was 82% and 82%, respectively. They compared these results with another group of patients that underwent resection whose 3- and 5-year survival was 48% and 21%, respectively. They concluded that liver transplantation achieves better survival with less recurrence than resection and that it should be considered an acceptable alternative to resection for HC. These conclusions are controversial and a thorough discussion of them is beyond the scope of this article because it is unclear how they apply to ICC. Nonetheless, at this time there seems to be no established role for liver transplantation outside of a clinical trial for ICC.

SURGICAL OUTCOMES
Survival

On examination of the more recent single institution series for resected patients with ICC, the 5-year survival has varied widely from 21% to 63% (**Table 1**). This is likely caused by differences in study methods because some included all resected patients, whereas others focused on R0 resected patients. Studies varied with respect to the number of patients with single or multiple tumors and the number of patients with locally advanced tumors.

Several studies have documented a trend toward improvement in overall survival over the last several decades in patients with ICC undergoing surgery.[17,18] Nathan and colleagues[28] used the SEER database to identify 591 patients with ICC who had undergone some form of cancer-directed surgery. When they compared the 5-year overall survival among the patients from 1973 to 1992 (N = 171 patients) with that of the 420 patients treated from 1993 to 2002, they found survival had increased from 16.5% to 22.9% ($P = .003$). They attributed the increase to improvements in patient selection with better imaging, and the more widespread use of hepatic resection from 1993 to 2002.

The authors recently reported a similar phenomenon at their institution where a marked increase in incidence in ICC was seen. When all patients presenting with a diagnosis of ICC from 1990 to 2006 were examined, the average annual incidence was found to increase by 14.2% (14 in 1990–1993 to 101 in 2003–2006). In total, 270 patients presented to Memorial Sloan-Kettering Cancer Center over this time period of whom 238 were subjected to outcomes analysis. Most of them were unresectable (68%), 128 determined by imaging and an additional 33 determined at exploration. Over time, the median survival for both the resected and unresected groups significantly improved. For the unresected group the median survival improved from 6 months (1990–2000) to 15 months (2001–2006) ($P = .003$). Likewise, for the resected group, the median survival from 1990 to 2000 was 33 months, whereas from 2001 to 2006 the median survival has not been reached ($P = .043$). The improvement in survival in the unresected group may be attributed to newer systemic agents and the application of regional chemotherapy to the liver. Improved survival seen in the resected patients also is likely caused by better patient selection.

Recurrence

Despite the apparent improvement in survival among resected patients over time, recurrence is still observed in most. In the authors' series of 82 resected patients,

Table 1
Comparison of recent surgical series in patients with intrahepatic cholangiocarcinoma

Author	Year	Patient Number	Number Resected	Resectability Rate (%)	3-Y Survival (Resected)	5-Y Survival (Resected)	Negative Prognostic Factors (Multivariate Analyses)
Harrison et al[49]	1998	32	32	NR	NR	42	Vascular invasion Multiple tumors
Weimann et al[50]	2000	162	95	59	31	21	Node positive Distant metastases Jaundice AJCC stage
Inoue et al[51]	2000	52	52	NR	NR	36	Positive margin Node positive Vascular invasion
Weber et al[15]	2001	53	33	62	22[a]	NR	Vascular invasion Multiple tumors Positive margin
Jan et al[52]	2004	373	135	36	9.2[b]	4.1[b]	Absence of mucobilia Nonpapillary histology No resection No postoperative chemotherapy
Lang et al[16]	2005	50	27	54	82 (R0)	NR	Positive margin Vascular invasion
Paik et al[35]	2007	97	97	NR	52	31	Positive margin Multiple tumors
DeOliveira et al[18]	2007	44	29	66	NR	63 (R0)	Positive margin Node positive

Study	Year						Prognostic factors
Nathan et al[53]	2007	591	NR	NR	NR	17%[b]	Age Regional and distant disease
Konstadoulakis et al[54]	2007	72	54	71%	49	25	None significant
Nakagohri et al[28]	2008	56	56	NR	NR	32	Multiple tumors
Tamandl et al[36]	2008	74	74	NR	45	28	Tumor size >5 cm Multiple tumors CA19-9 >100 UICC stage
Endo et al[17]	2008	238	77	32	NR	NR	Multiple tumors Lymph node positive Tumor size >5 cm

NR, not reported.
[a] Disease-free survival.
[b] Unresected + resected.

51 (62%) had recurred at a median follow-up of 26 months. The liver was the most common site of recurrence either alone or in combination with some extrahepatic site (32 [62.7%] of 51). Factors that most influenced recurrence were the number of tumors (solitary versus multiple) and the presence of lymph node metastases. In patients with solitary tumors with no lymph node metastases, the recurrence rate was 47%, whereas it increased to 93% when patients had multiple tumors or lymph node metastases.

Nakagohri and colleagues[29] reported recurrence in 31 (55%) of 56 patients resected and included the location of recurrences. The most common sites of recurrence were the liver,[18] hepatic hilus,[14] peritoneum,[7] and para-aortic lymph nodes.[5] The high number of recurrences in the hepatic hilus is interesting because this was not the finding by Shimada and colleagues,[20] where they found 23 patients recurred among 49 resected with none in the portal lymph nodes. The high rate of recurrence and high number of intrahepatic recurrences suggest that liver-directed adjuvant therapy may be a logical approach.

Prognostic Variables

There are a multitude of variables that have been found to correlate with survival among the studies in surgery for ICC. The most common seem to be multiple versus single tumors, lymph node metastases, and margin status.

Multiple hepatic tumors

This variable, more than any other, has been found to be an independent predictor of poor outcome. The presence of multiple tumors is believed to represent intrahepatic metastases and is often referred to as "multifocal disease." The outcomes of patients undergoing resection for multifocal disease have been so poor that most argue that this should be a contraindication to resection. In the authors' series of 82 resections, multiple intrahepatic tumors were found to be the only factor that was an independent predictor of both disease-specific and disease-free survival (**Fig. 3**).[17] The median

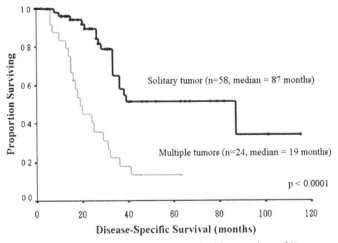

Fig. 3. Disease-specific survival after resection, stratified by number of liver tumors: solitary (*black line*, N = 58 months, median = 87 months) versus multiple (*gray line*, N = 24, median = 19 months); P<.0001. (*From* Endo I, Gonen M, Yopp AC, et al. Intrahepatic cholangiocarcinoma: rising frequency, improved survival, and determinants of outcome after resection. Ann Surg 2008;248:84–96; with permission.)

survival of the resected patients with multifocal disease was no different than the patients with liver-only disease that were treated nonoperatively.

Nakagohri and colleagues[29] found that no patient with multifocal disease survived beyond 10 months after resection. In their multivariate analysis the relative risk of death for multifocal disease was 5.38, well above the relative risk of any other variable. In light of all of these results, the authors do not advocate resection in patients with multifocal disease. Recently, it has been their practice to offer systemic or hepatic arterial infusional chemotherapy to these patients on clinical trials.

Lymph node metastases

This variable is the second most commonly reported independent predictor of outcome in resection for ICC. In the authors' series of 82 resected patients they performed a lymph node dissection or sampling in 55% and found 7 patients to have portal lymph node metastases. The median survival for these seven patients was 7 months versus 16 months for patients without lymph node metastases $(P = .012)$.[17]

Some have questioned the indication for surgery in patients with ICC and portal node involvement. Uenishi and colleagues[30] attempted to clarify this issue through a retrospective review of 145 patients who underwent curative hepatic resection for ICC in addition to portal lymphadenectomy. The extent of lymphadenectomy for all patients consisted of nodes along the hepatoduodenal ligament (group 1); nodes along the hepatic, celiac, and left gastric arteries (group 2); or para-aortic nodes (group 3). Twelve patients died perioperatively leaving 133 subject to survival analysis. Patients with a solitary tumor and no lymph node involvement had the best survival. Patients with multifocal disease and negative lymph nodes and patients with a solitary tumor and positive lymph node involvement had an intermediate survival. The survival of patients with multifocal disease and lymph node metastases was the worst (**Fig. 4**).

There is no current consensus on the value (either for staging or therapeutic purposes) of routine portal lymphadenectomy. It is clear that the presence of portal lymph node metastases is a poor prognostic variable and a sign of advanced disease.

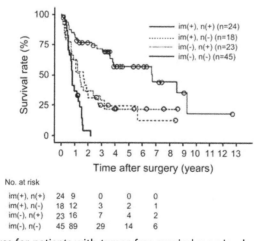

Fig. 4. Survival curves for patients with tumor-free surgical margins, based on lymph node metastases and intrahepatic metastases. im, intrahepatic metastases; n, lymph node metastases; (+), positive; (−), negative. (*From* Uenishi T, Kubo S, Yamazaki O, et al. Indications for surgical treatment of intrahepatic cholangiocarcinoma with lymph node metastases. J Hepatobiliary Pancreat Surg 2008;15:417–22; with permission.)

There are, however, a number of cases reported of long-term survivors with lymph node metastases.[31–33] In addition, two reports from Japan have argued for a therapeutic benefit to lymph node dissection when there is a solitary hepatic tumor and only one or two metastatic lymph nodes.[34,35] The authors believe portal lymph node metastases to be a sufficiently poor prognostic feature that they would exercise severe caution in resecting in patients whom are suspected either preoperatively or intraoperatively to have portal node involvement. The authors do not, however, consider this to be an absolute contraindication to resection.

Margin status
There is controversy in the literature as to the impact of a positive margin on survival after resection for ICC. Several reports have documented it as an independent predictor of survival on multivariate analyses.[15,16,19,36] Alternatively, several reports have not found margin status to be a statistically significant predictor of outcome. In their series of 82 resections the authors did not find margin status to be a statistically significant predictor of either disease-free or disease-specific survival.

The impact of surgical margins on recurrence and survival and the optimal width of margin were recently studied for ICC. Tamandl and colleagues[37] reported a series of 74 patients who underwent curative resection for ICC. There were 15 R1 resections and they stratified the remaining 59 R0 resections by margin widths of greater than 10 mm and 1 to 10 mm. They found that margin status (R0 versus R1) was not an independent predictor of either recurrence-free or overall survival. Among the 47 patients with recurrence (70%) they found that patients with a close margin (1–10 mm) or a positive margin did not experience more hepatic recurrences, nor did they have a different distribution of recurrences (hepatic versus extrahepatic) than patients with a wide margin (>10 mm). They concluded that there is no benefit to a wider margin. The authors attributed their findings to the application of a vaporizing ultrasonic dissection device that they routinely use to divide the liver parenchyma since 2000. This device reportedly can ablate tissue up to 5 mm from cut liver surface.[38]

Although the evidence supporting the importance of a negative surgical margin on outcome is not overwhelming, there are sufficient data to justify making a negative surgical margin the goal for every resection. The size of the margin does not seem to matter.

ADJUVANT THERAPY

The role of adjuvant therapy in patients with cholangiocarcinoma of all types is controversial. Because of the poor response of cholangiocarcinomas to cytotoxic chemotherapy and to the relative rarity of these tumors, there are no data to support its use in the adjuvant setting. The use of external beam radiation in the adjuvant setting is also controversial. Most of the studies have focused on patients with HC where its benefit is also questionable.

One study has focused on patients with ICC comparing surgery plus radiation with surgery alone. This study demonstrated a better overall survival in the surgery and radiation group (median survival surgery plus radiation 11 months versus 6 months surgery alone; $P = .0138$).[39] This study is questionable because it is a retrospective comparison from the SEER database and very little is known about the stage of disease, the extent of surgery, or the final pathology. In addition, the median survival in the surgery-alone group is well below that of most current series of resected patients.

At this time the authors do not advocate routine adjuvant systemic chemotherapy or radiation therapy in patients with ICC who have undergone a complete resection. Given the high recurrence rates, however, it is reasonable to consider adjuvant therapies in selected circumstances. Clinical trials are desperately needed to define the role of these therapies.

NONSURGICAL MANAGEMENT

Most patients with ICC present with unresectable disease. Survival in untreated patients is reported to be only 5 to 8 months.[40] Treatment options for these patients consist of systemic or regional chemotherapy, transarterial chemoembolization (TACE), external beam radiation, and thermal ablation. None of these modalities has any proved efficacy over best supportive care or over one another.

Systemic chemotherapy has improved from traditional 5-FU–based regimens that had response rates of only 10% to 30% to gemcitabine-based regimens with response rates in the range of 22% to 36%.[41] Regional chemotherapy has also been studied in primary liver cancer including ICC and has shown response rates in the range of 40% to 45% and median survival times up to 14 months.[42–45] This modality is generally reserved for patients with liver-only disease.

TACE is a treatment modality with proved efficacy in two randomized trials in patients with unresectable hepatocellular carcinoma;[46,47] however, data regarding of the use of TACE in unresectable ICC are limited to small retrospective studies. Gusani and colleagues[48] reported one of the largest studies to date of TACE in unresectable ICC consisting of 42 patients treated with one of five gemcitabine-based regimens. Patients were first given an infusion of chemotherapy to either the left or right hemiliver, followed by embolization. The median number of TACE treatments per patient was 3.5. TACE was relatively well tolerated with no mortality, five patients with grade 3, and two patients with grade 4 adverse events. Median overall survival from the time of the first TACE was 9.1 months. They found differences in survival between the gemcitabine-alone regimen and the combination regimen of gemcitabine-cisplatin (6.3 months versus 13.8 months; $P = .0005$).

The role of radiation in patients with ICC is poorly defined. Studies vary with respect to patient populations (unresected and resected patients); location of the disease (ICC versus HC); and the type of radiation delivered (external beam versus brachytherapy). A recent Chinese study focused on patients with unresectable ICC.[49] This was a case-control study that had among 38 patients in the radiotherapy group 22 who had unresectable ICC. These patients received a median total dose of 50 Gy in daily doses of 2 Gy per fraction, five times a week. Objective responses in the 22 unresectable ICC patients were observed in 36.4%. Pain was relieved in 90%. The survival rate at 1 and 2 years for the treated group (N = 22) was 36% and 19% versus 5.2% and 4.7% for the untreated group (N = 23) ($P = .021$).

In patients with small tumors away from major vascular or biliary structures who are not candidates for resection (because of poor liver function or comorbidities) thermal ablation is a reasonable option. There are many percutaneous and laparoscopic approaches that use cryotherapy, radiofrequency ablation, or microwave ablation with proved efficacy in many tumors. Thermal ablation for ICC is minimally studied.

SUMMARY

ICC remains a relatively poorly understood malignancy despite its recent rise in incidence in the United States. Although there has not been a randomized trial comparing surgery with other nonsurgical treatments, the standard of care has evolved through empiric data to consist of surgical resection when complete tumor removal can be achieved. This includes extended parenchymal or biliary and vascular resections when necessary provided they can be performed safely. Results of resection in the presence of multifocal disease have been poor enough such that resection is not recommended. Patients with portal lymph node metastases also have poor outcomes and extreme caution should be exercised in considering resection for these patients. Controversy exists regarding the role for adjuvant therapy after resection and prospective trials are needed. Several nonsurgical treatment modalities are available for unresectable patients, although some are only available at specialized centers.

REFERENCES

1. Malhi H, Gores GJ. Cholangiocarcinoma: modern advances in understanding a deadly old disease. J Hepatol 2006;45(6):856–67.
2. Patel T. Increasing incidence and mortality of primary intrahepatic cholangiocarcinoma in the United States. Hepatology 2001;33(6):1353–7.
3. Taylor-Robinson SD, Foster GR, Arora S, et al. Increase in primary liver cancer in the UK, 1979–94. Lancet 1997;350(9085):1142–3.
4. Kato I, Kuroishi T, Tominaga S. Descriptive epidemiology of subsites of cancers of the liver, biliary tract and pancreas in Japan. Jpn J Clin Oncol 1990;20(3):232–7.
5. Shin HR, Lee CU, Park HJ, et al. Hepatitis B and C virus, *Clonorchis sinensis* for the risk of liver cancer: a case-control study in Pusan, Korea. Int J Epidemiol 1996;25(5):933–40.
6. Su WC, Chan KK, Lin XZ, et al. A clinical study of 130 patients with biliary tract cancers and periampullary tumors. Oncology 1996;53(6):488–93.
7. Tan JC, Coburn NG, Baxter NN, et al. Surgical management of intrahepatic cholangiocarcinoma: a population-based study. Ann Surg Oncol 2008;15(2):600–8.
8. Miller G, Schwartz LH, D'Angelica M. The use of imaging in the diagnosis and staging of hepatobiliary malignancies. Surg Oncol Clin N Am 2007;16(2): 343–68.
9. Manfredi R, Barbaro B, Masselli G, et al. Magnetic resonance imaging of cholangiocarcinoma. Semin Liver Dis 2004;24(2):155–64.
10. Maetani Y, Itoh K, Watanabe C, et al. MR imaging of intrahepatic cholangiocarcinoma with pathologic correlation. AJR Am J Roentgenol 2001;176(6):1499–507.
11. Nichols JC, Gores GJ, LaRusso NF, et al. Diagnostic role of serum CA19-9 for cholangiocarcinoma in patients with primary sclerosing cholangitis. Mayo Clin Proc 1993;68(9):874–9.
12. Kim YJ, Yun M, Lee WJ, et al. Usefulness of 18F-FDG PET in intrahepatic cholangiocarcinoma. Eur J Nucl Med Mol Imaging 2003;30(11):1467–72.
13. Petrowsky H, Wildbrett P, Husarik DB, et al. Impact of integrated positron emission tomography and computed tomography on staging and management of gallbladder cancer and cholangiocarcinoma. J Hepatol 2006;45(1):43–50.
14. Goere D, Wagholikar GD, Pessaux P, et al. Utility of staging laparoscopy in subsets of biliary cancers: laparoscopy is a powerful diagnostic tool in patients with intrahepatic and gallbladder carcinoma. Surg Endosc 2006;20(5):721–5.
15. Weber SM, Jarnagin WR, Klimstra D, et al. Intrahepatic cholangiocarcinoma: resectability, recurrence pattern, and outcomes. J Am Coll Surg 2001;193(4): 384–91.
16. Lang H, Sotiropoulos GC, Fruhauf NR, et al. Extended hepatectomy for intrahepatic cholangiocellular carcinoma (ICC): when is it worthwhile? Single center experience with 27 resections in 50 patients over a 5-year period. Ann Surg 2005;241(1):134–43.

17. Endo I, Gonen M, Yopp AC, et al. Intrahepatic cholangiocarcinoma: rising frequency, improved survival, and determinants of outcome after resection. Ann Surg 2008;248(1):84–96.
18. DeOliveira ML, Cunningham SC, Cameron JL, et al. Cholangiocarcinoma: thirty-one-year experience with 564 patients at a single institution. Ann Surg 2007; 245(5):755–62.
19. Nakagohri T, Asano T, Kinoshita H, et al. Aggressive surgical resection for hilar-invasive and peripheral intrahepatic cholangiocarcinoma. World J Surg 2003; 27(3):289–93.
20. Shimada M, Yamashita Y, Aishima S, et al. Value of lymph node dissection during resection of intrahepatic cholangiocarcinoma. Br J Surg 2001;88(11):1463–6.
21. Grobmyer SR, Wang L, Gonen M, et al. Perihepatic lymph node assessment in patients undergoing partial hepatectomy for malignancy. Ann Surg 2006; 244(2):260–4.
22. Meyer CG, Penn I, James L. Liver transplantation for cholangiocarcinoma: results in 207 patients. Transplantation 2000;69(8):1633–7.
23. Shimoda M, Farmer DG, Colquhoun SD, et al. Liver transplantation for cholangio-cellular carcinoma: analysis of a single-center experience and review of the literature. Liver Transpl 2001;7(12):1023–33.
24. Goss JA, Shackleton CR, Farmer DG, et al. Orthotopic liver transplantation for primary sclerosing cholangitis: a 12-year single center experience. Ann Surg 1997;225(5):472–81 [discussion: 81–3].
25. Broome U, Olsson R, Loof L, et al. Natural history and prognostic factors in 305 Swedish patients with primary sclerosing cholangitis. Gut 1996;38(4):610–5.
26. Ghali P, Marotta PJ, Yoshida EM, et al. Liver transplantation for incidental cholangiocarcinoma: analysis of the Canadian experience. Liver Transpl 2005;11(11): 1412–6.
27. Rea DJ, Heimbach JK, Rosen CB, et al. Liver transplantation with neoadjuvant chemoradiation is more effective than resection for hilar cholangiocarcinoma. Ann Surg 2005;242(3):451–8 [discussion: 8–61].
28. Nathan H, Pawlik TM, Wolfgang CL, et al. Trends in survival after surgery for cholangiocarcinoma: a 30-year population-based SEER database analysis. J Gastrointest Surg 2007;11(11):1488–96 [discussion: 96–7].
29. Nakagohri T, Kinoshita T, Konishi M, et al. Surgical outcome and prognostic factors in intrahepatic cholangiocarcinoma. World J Surg 2008;32(12): 2675–80.
30. Uenishi T, Kubo S, Yamazaki O, et al. Indications for surgical treatment of intrahepatic cholangiocarcinoma with lymph node metastases. J Hepatobiliary Pancreat Surg 2008;15(4):417–22.
31. Asakura H, Ohtsuka M, Ito H, et al. Long-term survival after extended surgical resection of intrahepatic cholangiocarcinoma with extensive lymph node metastasis. Hepatogastroenterology 2005;52(63):722–4.
32. Murakami Y, Yokoyama T, Takesue Y, et al. Long-term survival of peripheral intrahepatic cholangiocarcinoma with metastasis to the para-aortic lymph nodes. Surgery 2000;127(1):105–6.
33. Yamamoto M, Takasaki K, Imaizumi T, et al. A long-term survivor of intrahepatic cholangiocarcinoma with lymph node metastasis: a case report. Jpn J Clin Oncol 2002;32(6):206–9.
34. Nakagawa T, Kamiyama T, Kurauchi N, et al. Number of lymph node metastases is a significant prognostic factor in intrahepatic cholangiocarcinoma. World J Surg 2005;29(6):728–33.

35. Suzuki S, Sakaguchi T, Yokoi Y, et al. Clinicopathological prognostic factors and impact of surgical treatment of mass-forming intrahepatic cholangiocarcinoma. World J Surg 2002;26(6):687–93.
36. Paik KY, Jung JC, Heo JS, et al. What prognostic factors are important for resected intrahepatic cholangiocarcinoma? J Gastroenterol Hepatol 2008;23(5):766–70.
37. Tamandl D, Herberger B, Gruenberger B, et al. Influence of hepatic resection margin on recurrence and survival in intrahepatic cholangiocarcinoma. Ann Surg Oncol 2008;15(10):2787–94.
38. Bodingbauer M, Tamandl D, Schmid K, et al. Size of surgical margin does not influence recurrence rates after curative liver resection for colorectal cancer liver metastases. Br J Surg 2007;94(9):1133–8.
39. Shinohara ET, Mitra N, Guo M, et al. Radiation therapy is associated with improved survival in the adjuvant and definitive treatment of intrahepatic cholangiocarcinoma. Int J Radiat Oncol Biol Phys 2008;72(5):1495–501.
40. Chou FF, Sheen-Chen SM, Chen YS, et al. Surgical treatment of cholangiocarcinoma. Hepatogastroenterology 1997;44(15):760–5.
41. Thongprasert S, Napapan S, Charoentum C, et al. Phase II study of gemcitabine and cisplatin as first-line chemotherapy in inoperable biliary tract carcinoma. Ann Oncol 2005;16(2):279–81.
42. Atiq OT, Kemeny N, Niedzwiecki D, et al. Treatment of unresectable primary liver cancer with intrahepatic fluorodeoxyuridine and mitomycin C through an implantable pump. Cancer 1992;69(4):920–4.
43. Cantore M, Rabbi C, Guadagni S, et al. Intra-arterial hepatic chemotherapy combined with continuous infusion of 5-fluorouracil in patients with metastatic cholangiocarcinoma. Ann Oncol 2002;13(10):1687–8.
44. Tanaka N, Yamakado K, Nakatsuka A, et al. Arterial chemoinfusion therapy through an implanted port system for patients with unresectable intrahepatic cholangiocarcinoma: initial experience. Eur J Radiol 2002;41(1):42–8.
45. Shitara K, Ikami I, Munakata M, et al. Hepatic arterial infusion of mitomycin C with degradable starch microspheres for unresectable intrahepatic cholangiocarcinoma. Clin Oncol (R Coll Radiol) 2008;20(3):241–6.
46. Llovet JM, Real MI, Montana X, et al. Arterial embolisation or chemoembolisation versus symptomatic treatment in patients with unresectable hepatocellular carcinoma: a randomised controlled trial. Lancet 2002;359(9319):1734–9.
47. Lo CM, Ngan H, Tso WK, et al. Randomized controlled trial of transarterial lipiodol chemoembolization for unresectable hepatocellular carcinoma. Hepatology 2002;35(5):1164–71.
48. Gusani NJ, Balaa FK, Steel JL, et al. Treatment of unresectable cholangiocarcinoma with gemcitabine-based transcatheter arterial chemoembolization (TACE): a single-institution experience. J Gastrointest Surg 2008;12(1):129–37.
49. Zeng ZC, Tang ZY, Fan J, et al. Consideration of the role of radiotherapy for unresectable intrahepatic cholangiocarcinoma: a retrospective analysis of 75 patients. Cancer J 2006;12(2):113–22.
50. Harrison LE, Fong Y, Klimstra DS, et al. Surgical treatment of 32 patients with peripheral intrahepatic cholangiocarcinoma. Br J Surg 1998;85(8):1068–70.
51. Weimann A, Varnholt H, Schlitt HJ, et al. Retrospective analysis of prognostic factors after liver resection and transplantation for cholangiocellular carcinoma. Br J Surg 2000;87(9):1182–7.

52. Inoue K, Makuuchi M, Takayama T, et al. Long-term survival and prognostic factors in the surgical treatment of mass-forming type cholangiocarcinoma. Surgery 2000;127(5):498–505.
53. Jan YY, Yeh CN, Yeh TS, et al. Prognostic analysis of surgical treatment of peripheral cholangiocarcinoma: two decades of experience at Chang Gung Memorial Hospital. World J Gastroenterol 2005;11(12):1779–84.
54. Konstadoulakis MM, Roayaie S, Gomatos IP, et al. Fifteen-year, single-center experience with the surgical management of intrahepatic cholangiocarcinoma: operative results and long-term outcome. Surgery 2008;143(3):366–74.

Surgical Management of Gallbladder Cancer

Srinevas K. Reddy, MD*, Bryan M. Clary, MD

KEYWORDS

- Gallbladder cancer • Management • Staging
- Incidence • Imaging

Relatively low disease incidence, high frequency of advanced, unresectable disease at initial presentation, nihilistic views of survival even after margin-negative surgical extirpation, and lack of established effective adjuvant therapy have all contributed to the absence of standardized surgical management of gallbladder cancer (GBCa). Aggressive tumor biology and a multitude of mechanisms of disease spread render 75% of preoperative suspected GBCa unresectable secondary to locally advanced or distant metastatic disease.[1] More than 80% of GBCa are adenocarcinomas,[2–4] which can be categorized into papillary, tubular, mucinous, and signet cell types.[5,6] GBCa can spread through lymphatic, hematogenous, transperitoneal, and neural mechanisms. Macroscopically, the tumor can spread by direct liver bed invasion or into the hilum along Glisson's sheath. Direct invasion into the liver is caused by short direct communicating veins that drain the gallbladder into segment IV (by the middle hepatic vein) or by veins accompanying extrahepatic ducts into the liver.[5] Transperitoneal spread can involve the liver, common bile duct, duodenum, pancreas, colon, or stomach and can manifest as peritoneal carcinomatosis in advanced stages.[5] The most common presenting symptoms include abdominal pain, biliary colic, and jaundice either from direct invasion of the biliary tree or nodal compression within the hepatoduodenal ligament.[1,7] Because of the rarity of GBCa, most patients are presumed to have benign disease and undergo subsequent operations that may violate tumor planes, complicating future attempts at oncologic resection. Furthermore, the nihilistic attitude of physicians prevents many patients from being offered an aggressive procedure to achieve an R0 resection. Even when an aggressive resection is used, the heterogeneity of accepted extirpative procedures (including anatomic or nonanatomic hepatic resections of segments 4b/5, right or extended right hepatectomy, formal portal lymphadenectomy, bile duct resection, pancreaticoduodenectomy, or resection of distant nodal disease) makes it difficult to assess the value of these extended resections. This article describes the epidemiology, risk factors, diagnostic imaging tools, and operative management of GBCa.

Department of Surgery, Duke University Medical Center, Box 3247, Durham, NC 27710, USA
* Corresponding author.
E-mail address: reddy005@mc.duke.edu (S.K. Reddy).

Surg Oncol Clin N Am 18 (2009) 307–324
doi:10.1016/j.soc.2008.12.004
1055-3207/08/$ – see front matter © 2009 Elsevier Inc. All rights reserved.

INCIDENCE AND EPIDEMIOLOGY

International and United States national registry data demonstrate substantial ethnic variability in the incidence of GBCa, with women affected more than men in most populations.[1,6] High incidences have been reported among women in Latin America (3.7–15.5 per 100,000);[6,8] native Americans in New Mexico (9.8–14.5 per 100,000);[6,9] women and men from East Asia (0.4%–0.6%);[10] Indian women (21.5 per 100,000);[11] and Pakistani women (13.8 per 100,000).[11] High rates were also noted in several cancer registries in Eastern Europe (Slovakia, Poland, Czech Republic, and Yugoslavia).[11] GBCa affects women two to six times more frequently than men; the extent of this difference varies and is greatest in regions with the highest rates of GBCa. As incidence decreases, the gender bias also decreases and approaches (but does not reach) parity.[8] A survey of 33 United States population-based registries during 1997 to 2002 revealed white men had a significantly lower age-adjusted incidence of GBCa compared with other racial-ethnic groups, with the highest rates among American Indian–Alaska natives and Asian–Pacific Islanders. Non-Hispanic men had significantly lower rates of GBCa than did Hispanic men. Similar racial and ethnic patterns of GBCa incidence were found among women, although the rate was highest among American Indian–Alaska natives. The incidence among Hispanics was more than twice than among non-Hispanics.[12] A gradual reduction in the per year incidence of the disease occurred over the last decade of study between 1993 and 2002 in both male and female patients, primarily in patients older than 50 years, when compared with patients diagnosed between 1973 and 1992.[12]

GALLSTONES AND GALLBLADDER CANCER

Although there is no direct evidence showing that gallstones cause GBCa, there are several theories linking GBCa to cholelithiasis. Gallstones can lead to gallbladder inflammation either by direct mechanical irritation to the surrounding mucosal surface or by altering gallbladder function leading to delayed or incomplete emptying with subsequent bile stasis and dilation of the gallbladder.[8] This inflammation may promote epithelial dysplastic and metaplastic changes leading to adenocarcinoma. It has been suggested that larger stones have a greater impact on the risk of developing GBCa, possibly reflecting greater duration and intensity of epithelial irritation.[6,8,13] Furthermore, cholelithiasis is considerably more frequent in patients with GBCa than in those with other types of biliary-tract cancer, providing further evidence that the inflammatory effects of cholelithiasis are important risk factors for GBCa.[8] Several case-control, cross-sectional, and cohort studies demonstrate a relationship between gallstones and GBCa across the world (**Table 1**). Summary of case-control and cohort studies demonstrated a relative risk for history of gallstones was 4.9 (95% confidence interval [CI], 3.3–7.4); 2.2 (95% CI, 1.2–4.2) among cohort studies; and 7.1 (95% CI, 4.5–11.2) among case-control studies with significant heterogeneity among all studies ($P<.001$).[6] In a comparison between 78 asymptomatic patients with cholelithiasis, 365 symptomatic patients with cholelithiasis, and 149 patients with GBCa, Csendes and colleagues[14] noted that patients with GBCa more often had multiple stones (more than 11) compared with the groups with asymptomatic and symptomatic gallstones ($P<.01$). Patients with GBCa had significantly larger stones compared with the other two groups, regardless of the number of stones present ($P<.001$).[14] Similarly, Roa and colleagues[15] note that the average number, weight, and volume of gallstones were higher among patients with GBCa compared with control patients with chronic cholecystitis.

Table 1				
Association of gallbladder cancer with gallstones				
Author	Site	Study Type	Population	Odds Ratio
Chow et al[16]	Denmark	Cohort	60,176	SIR 4.6 (3.0–6.7) (1–4 y follow-up) SIR 2.7 (1.5–4.4) (≥5-y follow-up)
Zatonski et al[17]	Australia, Canada, Netherlands, Poland	Case-control	1711	4.4 (2.6–7.5)
Okamoto et al[18]	Japan	Cross-sectional	194,767	$P<.01$
Kimura et al[19]	Japan	Cross-sectional	4482	$P<.01$
Nervi et al[20]	Chile	Cross-sectional	14,768	7, $P<.05$
Maringhini et al[21]	United States	Cross-sectional	2583	$P<.05$ in men
Ishiguro et al[22]	Japan	Cohort	101,868	3.10 (1.55–6.19)
Hsing et al[23]	China	Cohort	2623	Family history: 2.1 (1.4–3.3) 21 (14.8–30.1); no family history of gallstones

Abbreviation: SIR, Standard incidence ratio.

POLYPS

Although there is no direct evidence of the adenoma-dysplasia-carcinoma sequence (as in colorectal cancer), there is indirect evidence of this relationship in GBCa. Dysplasia and carcinoma in situ are found in the gallbladder mucosa adjacent to most carcinomas.[6] Yamagiwa[24] examined 110 cases of resected GBCa and found dysplasia adjacent to carcinoma in 46 of the 110 cases; this change was frequently found in lesions at an early stage and in well-differentiated carcinoma. In addition, patients with dysplasia and carcinoma in situ are 15 and 5 years younger, respectively, than those with invasive carcinoma, suggesting a temporal and progressive sequence.[6] Polyps suspicious for possible malignant transformation include those that are sessile, solitary, and greater than 1 cm in diameter; contrast enhancing on CT; or have visible blood supply on ultrasound (US).[5] Standard treatment for these patients is laparoscopic cholecystectomy. With highly suspicious lesions, however, open exploration, intraoperative frozen section, and preparation for extended resection should be undertaken.[5] Patients with fewer than three polyps, regardless of size, should undergo cholecystectomy, whereas patients with more than three polyps are likely to have pseudotumors, which can be observed if continued to be asymptomatic. For low-risk polyps, 6-month surveillance US is recommended for 2 years.[5]

IMAGING
Ultrasound

US patterns of GBCa include (1) the gallbladder is replaced by a mass of variable echogenicity filling the entire lumen with gallstones, air, or necrosis causing central echogenicity; (2) thickening of the gallbladder wall that can be diffuse or focal and hyperechoic or hypoechoic; and (3) an intraluminal mass with fungating appearance, irregular border, and variable echogenicity.[1,25] When the tumor grows as a mass occupying the gallbladder or gallbladder fossa, the lesion is hypoechoic or isoechoic with respect to the liver and is irregularly shaped because of infiltration of the neighboring hepatic parenchyma.[26] Importantly, these US findings do not provide reliable differentiation between a carcinoma and other nonneoplastic lesions, such as cholesterol polyps or adenomyomatosis.[26] Among 203 patients with histologically confirmed GBCa, US revealed a mass lesion in the gallbladder in 177 patients (87%). US was highly accurate in demonstrating gallbladder masses, gallstones, liver infiltration, and ascites. Although US may be useful in ascertaining the presence of portal vein or hepatic artery invasion,[1] it is not accurate for assessing common bile duct infiltration, lymph node involvement (especially pericholedochal and peripancreatic nodes), and peritoneal disease.[27] US is a good screening technique that may raise suspicion for GBCa, but other imaging studies should be used to confirm the presence of this disease and to define resectability better.

CT

On CT, GBCa can present as (1) a low-attenuation mass with variable enhancement reflective of scattered regions of internal necrosis that fills most of an enlarged and deformed gallbladder, (2) polypoid masses greater than 1 cm, and (3) symmetric or an asymmetric gallbladder wall thickening that may be difficult to distinguish from the scarred gallbladder wall seen in chronic cholecystitis.[25,26,28] Protrusion of the quadrate lobe with lymphadenopathy has also been reported to be unique to GBCa.[25] CT is also useful in defining resectability by detecting lymphatic spread, infiltration into hepatic parenchyma, bile ducts, or other neighboring organs, and peritoneal metastases. Infiltrated lymph nodes usually have an anteroposterior diameter of greater than 1 cm and are ring-shaped with heterogeneous uptake after contrast administration.[26]

Several studies have demonstrated excellent accuracy for CT in staging GBCa. In a study of 118 patients who were pathologically shown to have GBCa, Kim and colleagues[29] note a sensitivity of CT in differentiating T1 versus T2 lesions, T2 versus T3 lesions, and T3 versus T4 lesions of 79.3%, 92.7%, and 100%, respectively. Corresponding specificities were 98.8%, 86%, and 100%, respectively ($P<.0001$). The overall accuracy for T staging was 83.9%. Overstaging and understaging occurred in 11 (9.3%) and 8 (6.8%) of 118 patients, respectively. In the 53 patients with multiplanar reconstruction images, the combined reading of the axial and multiplanar reconstruction images increased the diagnostic accuracy compared with axial image reading only from 71.7% to 84.9% ($P = .0233$).[29] Among 21 patients with GBCa, helical CT provided 83% to 86% accuracy in the diagnosis of the local extent of carcinomas of the gallbladder, showing acceptable sensitivity and specificity for the T2 and more advanced lesions but poor sensitivity for the T1 lesions.[30] Among 100 patients with GBCa, the overall accuracy of CT staging of GBCa was 71%, 79% for T1 and T2 tumors, 46% for T3 tumors, and 73% for T4 tumors. Of 20 patients who presented to a single institution, CT had a sensitivity of 72.7%, a specificity of 100%, and an accuracy of 85% for determining resectability. There was 100% correlation between CT and surgery in diagnosing hepatic and vascular invasion.[31] Rao and colleagues[32] point out that magnetic resonance cholangiography did not provide additional information above that provided by three-dimensional helical CT in demonstrating the presence, site, and extent of biliary obstruction by GBCa in 25 consecutive patients.

Positron Emission Tomography

Theoretical benefits of positron emission tomography (PET) for GBCa include diagnosing otherwise ambiguous lesions, detecting residual disease after cholecystectomy, and in unmasking distant disease not detected by other imaging modalities.[1] Problems related to coexisting inflammation resulting in increased glucose metabolism could, however, confound the results in some patients. This limitation is important to recognize, because most patients with GBCa are diagnosed after undergoing cholecystectomy and often have varying degrees of postoperative inflammation.[33] Patients theoretically most likely to benefit from preoperative PET are those with evidence of increased tracer activity in regional lymph nodes, peritoneum, or other extra-abdominal sites suggesting metastatic disease for which resection is contraindicated.[33]

The data on PET for GBCa are comprised of small series that show that PET does not change operative management for most patients with GBCa. In a combined study with cholangiocarcinoma, Petrowsky and colleagues[34] show that PET-CT detected all GBCa (14 of 14), whereas CT alone identified the tumor in 10 (71%) of 14 patients ($P = .10$). All distant metastases (12 of 12) were detected by PET-CT, but only 3 of 12 by CT alone ($P<.001$), suggesting an added use of PET compared with CT alone. PET-CT findings resulted in a change of management, however, in only 17% of patients deemed resectable after standard work-up.[34] Among nine patients with residual GBCa after initial cholecystectomy (total of 14 patients), the sensitivity of PET for residual gallbladder carcinoma was 78% (seven of nine) and specificity was 80% (four of five). Sensitivity for extrahepatic metastases (distant metastases or carcinomatosis) was 56% (five of nine). PET detected intra-abdominal metastases in only three of six patients with confirmed carcinomatosis.[35] In another retrospective study, PET changed operative management in 7 (23%) of 31 patients by showing metastatic disease not seen on other imaging studies, thereby preventing an unnecessary exploration. The sensitivity of PET for GBCa was 86% for detecting the primary tumor or residual disease in the operative bed (in postcholecystectomy patients) and was 87% for detecting metastatic disease.[33]

MRI

Several studies have described the characteristic imaging qualities of GBCa on MRI.[25,26,36] The primary tumor is hypointense on T1 images and hyperintense or heterogeneous on T2 images compared with liver parenchyma. There is early, heterogeneous, and preferentially peripheral enhancement, which tends to progress slowly in a centripetal manner.[25] The outer uptake margin correlates well with the extent of the tumor, which is of particular value in assessing complete penetration of serosa or invasion of liver. MRI with magnetic resonance cholangiography and magnetic resonance angiography may also reveal invasion into the peritoneum, bile ducts, vessels, and duodenum or liver metastases and biliary obstruction.[25] In a study comprising 18 patients with resected GBCa, a combination of preoperative MRI, magnetic resonance angiography, and magnetic resonance cholangiography the sensitivity and specificity of MRI examination were 100% and 89% for bile duct invasion, 100% and 87% for vascular invasion, 67% and 89% for hepatic invasion, and 56% and 89% for lymph node metastasis.[37]

STAGING

There are several different staging criteria for GBCa. According to American Joint Committee on Cancer (AJCC) sixth edition TNM staging guidelines, T1 tumors invade the gallbladder lamina propria or muscle layers; T2 lesions invade perimuscular connective tissue without extension into liver; T3 tumors perforate visceral peritoneum or directly invade the liver or one other adjacent organ; and T4 carcinomas invade the main portal vein, hepatic artery, or multiple extrahepatic organs.[38] Any nodal disease is designated as N1 and distant metastatic disease is designated as M1. Stage I disease includes node-negative T1 or T2 disease, stage II disease includes any T3 and T1 to 3 node-positive disease, stage III includes any T4 disease, and stage IV includes any M1 disease.

In an analysis of the National Cancer Database, Fong and colleagues[39] propose an alternative staging system to the AJCC sixth edition in which stage II disease is only for T2N0M0 disease (as opposed to stage IIA for T3N0M0 disease and stage IIB for T1_3N1M0 disease in AJCC). In addition, increased emphasis is placed on nodal disease because nodal disease in the hepatoduodenal ligament is categorized as stage IIIB (for T1_3) or stage IVB (for T4) disease. This is in contrast to stage IIB and III, respectively, for the AJCC sixth edition staging. Moreover, nodal disease in the peripancreatic, periduodenal, periportal, celiac, or superior mesenteric nodes (N2) is classified as stage IVB disease and equivalent to distant metastases. In analyzing outcomes for 7462 patients who underwent potentially curative surgical therapy for GBCa, the authors argue that this proposed staging system better discriminates long-term outcomes between patients with stage II and stage III and between stage III and stage IV disease compared with the AJCC sixth edition. The Japanese Biliary Surgical Society staging system separates tumors into stage 1, cancers confined to the gallbladder capsule; stage 2, cancers with positive N1 lymph nodes or minimal liver–bile duct invasion; stage 3, positive N2 lymph nodes or marked liver–bile duct invasion; and stage 4, distant metastases. The original Nevin classification categorized patients into stage 1, in situ cancer; stage 2, cancer not yet transmural; stage 3, transmural direct liver invasion; stage 4, lymph node metastases; and stage 5, distant metastases.[39]

OPERATIVE INTERVENTION

Long-term survival after resection of GBCa is largely based on results of large, retrospective surgical extirpation series (**Table 2**). The marked heterogeneity in study sizes, procedures performed to obtain negative resection margins, and long-term survival reflects the absence of a standard for "resectable disease." Despite these study differences, tumor thickness (reflected in T stage), nodal disease, resection margin, and age were common variables associated with survival.

Incidental Disease

The frequency of incidental GBCa detected in histopathologic examination after cholecystectomy for presumed benign disease ranges from 0.27% to 2.1%.[40–42] In patients in whom the diagnosis is made intraoperatively by a surgeon not prepared to do a hepatic resection or bile duct reconstruction, the patient should be transferred to a medical center with hepatobiliary surgical expertise.[1] Several studies demonstrate that a previous cholecystectomy does not affect survival after definitive surgical extirpation.[43–46] Fong and colleagues[2] show that previous surgical resection (most often simple cholecystectomy) did not lower the likelihood of a subsequent curative resection or impact overall survival on multivariable analysis for all 102 curative resections. Analysis of the Connecticut Tumor Registry data demonstrated that previous laparoscopic manipulation of a GBCa did not significantly affect survival, incidence of abdominal wall recurrences, or bile spillage.[47] Similarly, Kwon and colleagues[41] show no significant difference in survival between those patients diagnosed with GBCa during or after laparoscopic cholecystectomy. In a study of 40 patients with stage 0 or I GBCa (23 treated with open cholecystectomy and 17 treated with laparoscopic cholecystectomy), Chan and colleagues[48] demonstrate no difference in tumor recurrence or overall survival after cholecystectomy (which was definitive surgical extirpation). In a case control study comparing 24 patients who underwent laparoscopic cholecystectomy with 40 case-matched controls who underwent open cholecystectomy, there was no difference in overall survival after cholecystectomy (5-year 35% each).[49] Among nine patients who underwent laparoscopic cholecystectomy compared with 11 patients who underwent open cholecystectomy, Sarli and colleagues[50] show no difference in overall survival ($P = .60$) or recurrence-free survival ($P = .90$). On multivariable analysis, tumor stage and bile spillage were associated with survival. Biliary spillage occurred with equal frequency with open and laparoscopic cholecystectomy.[50] Toyonaga and colleagues[51] show that the type of initial cholecystectomy (open versus laparoscopic) did not influence survival.

Extended Cholecystectomy

The frequency of regional nodal disease is higher with thicker tumors as compared with T1 lesions. In a multi-institutional study of six major hepatobiliary centers, increasing T stage was associated with risk of finding any residual disease on reresection after initial cholecystectomy (T1 38%, T2 57%, T3 77%; $P = .01$); residual liver disease (T1 0%, T2 10%, T3 36%; $P = .006$); and risk of locoregional lymph node metastases (T1 13%, T2 31%, T3 46%; $P = .04$).[45] Similarly, Kai and colleagues[67] note that lymphatic, venous, and perineural invasion increase with increasing T stage. For T2 disease, rates were 81%, 53%, and 32%; for T3 disease rates were 75%, 100%, and 50%. The rates of lymph node involvement were 47% in T2, 62% in T3, and 69% in T4 disease. Other studies have noted a similar relationship between tumor thickness and regional nodal disease.[2,52,64]

Whereas a simple cholecystectomy is sufficient for T1 disease, most studies show that an extended cholecystectomy is necessary for long-term survival for T2 and T3 disease. Patients with T2 or T3 disease require a minimum of extended cholecystectomy for definitive extirpation because positive margins are noted after cholecystectomy in up to 24% of specimens and the incidence of lymph node involvement (39%–54%), and lymphatic, perineural, and venous invasion is high.[5] Extended cholecystectomy involves wedge resection of segments IVb and V to at least 3 cm depth from the gallbladder bed with regional lymphadenectomy (including nodes around the cystic duct, portal vein, hepatoduodenal ligament, and liver hilum).[5] In a small study, eight patients with T1 or Tis disease had no disease recurrence and 100% survival without reresection after cholecystectomy. In contrast, 8 of 14 patients with T2 tumors died. Patients who underwent reresection and lymphadenectomy (N = 7) had improved survival compared with patients who did not ($P = .027$).[42] Kwon and colleagues[41] note that 19 patients with T1 disease had a median survival of 68 months after laparoscopic cholecystectomy without additional resection. In a South Korean study of 75 patients of which 16% had nodal disease, Kang and colleagues[68] demonstrate as T stage increased, the incidence of R0 resection decreased. No patients with T1 disease died during follow-up and 5-year overall survival for T2 disease was 78%. In contrast, 5-year survival for T3 disease was 15%.[68] Toyonaga and colleagues[51] note that among 22 patients with incidental T1 disease, none underwent subsequent radical resection and there was no evidence of recurrence during follow-up. A total of 37% and 100% of patients with T2 and T3 disease developed disease recurrence, despite subsequent radical resection in 42% of patients. Subsequent radical resection only improved survival for patients with T2 disease in those with positive resection margins at initial cholecystectomy, not those patients with negative margins.[51] Analysis of the German Society of Surgery registry of "incidental gallbladder carcinoma"

Table 2
Outcomes of large retrospective curative resection series for gallbladder cancer

Author	N	Age (y)	Survival	Predictors of Survival	Comments
Ito et al[52]	18	Median 66 (37–96)	1-y 73% 5-y 31%	Nodal disease Age >65 y	50% T2, 28% nodal disease Positive margin in 22% Probability of nodal disease increase with tumor thickness
Ruckert et al[53]	81	Mean 57 (50–60)	5-y 9%	Nodal disease Liver resection	65% stage IV, 78% nodal disease
Behari et al[54]	18	—	Median 25.8 mo	Nodal disease[a]	72% stage III
Fong et al[2]	100	Median 65	Median 26 mo 5-y 38%	Nodal disease T stage	42% extended resection
Shirai et al[55]	40	—	—	Nodal disease	5-y 85% for patients with or without nodal disease 5-y 45% for patients with nodal disease
Cubertafond et al[3]	724	Mean 69	5-y 5%	T stage	81% nodal disease 32% T3 and 53% T4 disease T1/T2 disease: median survival 22 mo
North et al[56]	36	Median 62	Median 67.2 mo 5-y 57%	T stage	All had R0 resection
Todoroki et al[57]	135	—	5-y 36%	Gender, T stage Nodal disease Margin status	66% T4 disease
Benoist et al[4]	86	—	1-y 63% 3-y 43% 5-y 26%	T stage Nodal disease	42% T1, 37% T2, 10% T3, 10% T4 66% underwent simple cholecystectomy

Study	N	Age	Survival	Stage, age, gender	
Kayahara et al[58]	3324	—	5-y men 37% / 5-y women 41%	Stage, age, gender	74% underwent curative resection / 66% R0 resection / Adjuvant chemotherapy did not impact survival except for stage IVA disease
Taner et al[44]	118	Median 65 (32–93)	5-y 21%[b]	AJCC stage / Radical resection	34% simple cholecystectomy, 45% radical resection / N1 33%, N2 24%, distant mets 30% of patients
Schauer et al[59]	45	Mean 66 (38–92)[a]	5-y 20% / Median 32.5 mo	Nodal status[a] / Grade[a]	—
Chan et al[60]	23	Median 70 (26–91)[a]	1-y 85% / 2-y 63% / 3-y 55% / 5-y 55%	—	Median DFS was 14 mo
Balachandran et al[61]	117	Median 53 (23–80)	5-y 27% / Median 16 mo	T status / Adjuvant Chemoradiotherapy / R0 resection	32% patients had a radical resection / 49% of radical resections had R0 resection / Radical resections improved survival for T3 tumors
Kokudo et al[62]	152	Mean 65 (41–86)	1-y 83% / 3-y 71% / 5-y 63%	T stage / Bile duct invasion	Bile duct resection did not improve survival / Extended lymph node dissection improved survival for patients with N2 disease
Kiran et al[12]	6421	Median 73	Median 22 mo (local disease) / Median 8 mo (regional disease)	More recent diagnosis	Adjuvant radiotherapy improved survival for regional disease (median 12 versus 6 mo, $P<.0001$)
Puhalla et al[63]	60	Mean 69.3	5-y 18.2%	R0 resection / Tumor grade	—

(continued on next page)

Table 2
(continued)

Author	N	Age (y)	Survival	Predictors of Survival	Comments
Yildirim et al[64]	65	Median 59 (34–77)	5-y 32% Median 41 mo	Nodal status R0 resection Extended resection[c]	All patients had initial cholecystectomy 5-y RFS 16% Frequency of positive nodes increases with T stage
Toyonaga et al[51]	73	Mean 65.7	—	T stage	Incidentally diagnosed after cholecystectomy 32% T1, 59% T2, 10% T3
Kohya and Miyazaki[65]	73	Mean 67.9	5-y 42%	Nodal status Liver and bile duct resection	5-y DFS 59%
Yagi et al[66]	63	Mean 66 (48–84)	—	Nodal disease High-density lipoprotein invasion Invasion of gallbladder bed	Stage I 36, stage II 11, stage III 6, stage IV 10 patients Liver resection associated with better survival for patients with disease not invading gallbladder bed Bile duct resection did not affect survival
Kai et al[67]	90	Mean 65 (36–89)	—	Nodal disease Portal vein invasion Surgical margin	17 T1, 34 T2, 9 T3, and 30 T4 patients

Abbreviations: AJCC, American Joint Committee on Cancer; DFS, Disease-free survival; RFS, Recurrence-free survival.
[a] For the entire series of patients (curative and noncurative resections).
[b] For those patients who underwent radical resection.
[c] For T2 and T3 stages.

reveals 439 cases, 200 of which are T2 tumors. A total of 21% and 44% of patients with T2 and T3 disease had positive nodal disease. Subsequent radical resection for T2 tumors was associated with improved survival (N = 85, 5-year 55% versus N = 115, 5-year 35%; P = .04). In contrast, there was no survival advantage for T3 tumors (P = .69). Long-term survival was only achievable if there was node-negative disease (P = .0078; 55% 5-year versus 0%) among patients with T2 tumors. There was no difference in survival among reresected patients who underwent IVb/V anatomic resections compared with hepatic wedge resections for patients with T2 disease (P = .34).[69] In a Japanese survey study of 498 patients who underwent initial laparoscopic cholecystectomy with GBCa, 34% of patients had T1a disease, 14% had T1b, 41% had T2, 8% had T3 disease, and 2% had T4 disease. Patients with T2 (P = .051) and T3 (P<.05) tumors had better survival with reresection compared with patients not reresected. There was no difference for T1 and T4 tumors.[70] In analysis of the Surveillance Epidemiology and End Results (SEER) database, radical resection (including resection of the gallbladder fossa and portal lymphadenectomy) for T1B/T2 tumors was associated with a significant improvement in cancer-specific (hazard ratio [HR] = 0.638 [0.430–0.949]; P = .0264) survival and a trend to improved overall survival (HR = 0.721 [0.517–1.006]; P = .0542) compared with simple cholecystectomy. Extended cholecystectomy was not associated with a survival benefit in patients with node-positive disease.[71] Benoist and colleagues[4] note no difference in survival between patients with T1a and T1b disease who underwent simple cholecystectomy, in contrast to those with T2 and T3 disease that did have worse survival compared with those with T1 disease. Radical cholecystectomy was associated with improved survival at every tumor stage except stage I.[44] Kai and colleagues[67] compared nine T2 patients who underwent simple cholecystectomy with 21 patients who underwent extended cholecystectomy; simple cholecystectomy was associated with worse survival (P = .0481). Similarly, portal lymph node resection (P = .0012) but not bile duct resection was associated with overall survival. Foster and colleagues[72] report the results of 64 patients who underwent resection for gallbladder GBCa. The 5-year survival was better for radical cholecystectomy versus simple cholecystectomy versus palliation (42% versus 22% versus 0%; P<.001). Of 38 patients with T2 or T3 disease, the survival after radical cholecystectomy (either as initial therapy or after initial simple cholecystectomy) was better than after simple cholecystectomy (median not reached, 5-year 62% versus median 17 months, 5-year 16%; P = .007).

Despite these data, extended cholecystectomy is rarely performed for patients with thick tumors. Analysis of 2835 patients in the SEER database revealed that resection of three or more lymph nodes (recommended by the AJCC for an adequate lymphadenectomy) was only obtained in 5.3% of patients.[73] T1 stage, relative to T2, (HR = 0.48, 0.27–0.83), age greater than 60 (HR = 0.42, 0.28–0.62), and year of resection (later than 1988, HR = 1.20, 1.14–1.26) were associated with lymphadenectomy (≥3 nodes resected). Lymphadenectomy was more likely to be performed in more recent resections, whereas it was less likely to be performed in older patients.[73] Further analysis of the SEER database showed that only 5.2% and 13.3% of patients with T2 and T3 disease underwent en bloc resection. Similarly, only 6.7% and 6% of patients with T2 and T3 disease underwent lymphadenectomy.[73] A total of 45% and 75% of all en bloc resections included either no or two or fewer lymph nodes. This implies that among the few patients where a more aggressive surgical resection was adopted, most patients did not undergo the oncologic standard extirpation for GBCa.[73] A second analysis of the SEER database for surgical management of 385 patients with T2 disease showed that only 4% (14 patients) underwent radical resection; the rest underwent simple cholecystectomy with or without lymphadenectomy.[74]

Bile duct resection
Resection of the extrahepatic bile duct has not been proved to improve survival for most patients with GBCa. Common bile duct resection is most often performed if the cystic duct stump margin from previous cholecystectomy was involved with tumor. In a multi-institutional study of six major hepatobiliary centers, 148 patients with incidental GBCa were treated with a single (N = 33) or two-staged operation (N = 115). Patients with a microscopically positive cystic duct stump margin (either on review of the initial pathology specimen or on biopsy of the cystic duct stump at time of reresection) were more likely to have disease in the common bile duct (42% versus 4%; $P = .01$).[45] There was no difference in number of lymph nodes harvested comparing portal lymphadenectomy alone with portal lymphadenectomy plus common bile duct resection (median 3, one to five, versus median 3, one to six; $P = .35$).[45] The extent of hepatectomy and common bile duct resection did not impact survival. On multivariable analysis, the stage of disease and the presence of residual cancer in the liver bed (not at the bile duct margin) both were associated with poor survival.[45] Sakamoto and colleagues[75] analyzed 87 patients with T2 to T4 disease who underwent extrahepatic bile duct resection. Survival of patients with ductal disease (N = 29) was less compared with patients without ductal disease (N = 58) (5-year survival 10% versus 55%; $P = .0001$). Of the latter group of patients, hepatic disease (HR = 4.82 [1.42–16.33]; $P = .01$) was the only factor independently associated with poor survival. There was no difference in the number of lymph nodes harvested between patients who did and did not undergo extrahepatic bile duct resection (median 13 [0–71] versus median 10 [0–38]; $P = .47$). There was no difference in survival among patients who underwent bile duct resection with or without lymph node metastases. Among patients with perineural invasion, those who underwent bile duct resection (N = 14) had improved survival compared with those who did not (N = 10) (5-year 46% versus 0%; $P = .0009$).

Extended hepatic resection
Although a radical cholecystectomy allows for an adequate margin near the gallbladder fundus, it results in a minimal margin at the base of the cystic plate and may not be sufficient for tumors that lie near the gallbladder neck, in Hartmann's pouch, or that extend into the triangle of Calot.[1] Isolated resection of segments IVb and V mandates preservation of the segment VIII branches of the right anterior portal pedicle. The proximity of the bifurcation of the anterior branch of the right portal vein to the gallbladder fossa poses an anatomic limitation to the extent of tumor clearance that can be achieved with a IVb/V resection.[73] Moreover in cases of previous cholecystectomy, the triangle of Calot is often obliterated by tumor or scar, making it difficult to distinguish cancer from benign inflammatory tissue. Because the plane of transection is well to the left of the cystic plate, extended hepatic resection may be especially useful in these patients as a sure method to achieve an oncologically negative resection margin by staying outside the plane of prior surgery. The authors typically perform an extended hepatectomy in the following circumstances: (1) when the cystic duct margin of the previous cholecystectomy specimen is positive or unknown; (2) after open cholecystectomy or when the initial operative indication is acute cholecystitis because it is anticipated that the triangle of Calot will be obliterated by scar tissue; (3) when node-positive disease is evident before hepatic resection (either in the initial cholecystectomy specimen or detected on preoperative imaging); (4) for patients presenting with preoperative jaundice caused by biliary obstruction; or (5) for large mass lesions detected on preoperative imaging (usually CT). Patients 75

years of age and older and those individuals with extensive medical comorbidity are typically not offered extended hepatectomy.[76]

The role of extended hepatectomy in decreasing local or regional disease recurrence and prolonging long-term survival compared with extended cholecystectomy is not well defined. Previously, the authors have reported experience with 11 patients with stage I (N = 2) or II (N = 9) disease who underwent major hepatic resection for gallbladder GBCa.[76] Indications for extended hepatectomy included large tumor size in patients who did not undergo previous simple cholecystectomy (N = 5); positive or unknown cystic duct margin status after simple cholecystectomy (N = 4); preoperative biliary obstruction (N = 1); known node-positive disease before hepatic resection (N = 4); and acute cholecystitis leading to simple cholecystectomy (N = 1). Of the 11 patients who underwent major hepatic resection, 5 (45%) of 11 are no evidence of disease (NED), 1 (9%) of 11 is alive with disease (AWD), and 5 (45%) of 11 are dead of disease (DOD) at last follow-up. All cases of first disease recurrence consisted of disseminated disease. Other investigators have reported similar results of isolated long-term survivors after extended hepatectomy.[76] Case-control comparative studies between extended hepatectomy and extended cholecystectomy, however, have not been performed.

Adjuvant therapy

Retrospective studies demonstrate a survival benefit to adjuvant radiotherapy for GBCa. In an analysis of the SEER database, 760 (18%) of 4180 patients were treated with adjuvant radiotherapy. Patients with more locally advanced (T2 or greater but without metastases) and node-positive disease were more likely to have received adjuvant radiotherapy. The unadjusted median overall survival time for patients who received radiotherapy was 15 months (95% CI, 13–16 months) compared with 8 months (95% CI, 8–9 months) for patients who did not receive radiotherapy ($P<.0001$). The association of adjuvant radiotherapy to survival remained significant on multivariable analysis (HR 1.46 [1.07–1.98]; $P = .014$). A multivariable Cox proportional hazards model was created to estimate which patients would benefit from adjuvant radiotherapy. For patients with T1 disease, the survival model estimated no survival benefit from postoperative radiotherapy regardless of nodal status. In contrast, the model predicted patients with higher stage ($\geq$T2), node-positive disease would derive the greatest benefit from adjuvant radiotherapy.[77] In a series of 85 patients with stage IV disease, Todoroki and colleagues[78] demonstrated that adjuvant radiation therapy improved long-term overall survival for patients who underwent R1 resection compared with no adjuvant therapy ($P = .0028$). Patients with R0 and R2 resections did not benefit from adjuvant therapy. In contrast, analysis of the Veteran Affairs Central Cancer Registry showed no difference in overall survival after resection of GBCa among patients who did and did not receive adjuvant chemotherapy (median 8.3 versus 8.7 months).[79] The authors have previously reported experience with adjuvant radiotherapy.[80] Of 22 patients (10 with node-positive disease) who underwent surgical extirpation, 18 received concurrent 5-fluorouracil. Median overall survival and disease-free survival were 1.9 and 1.6 years, respectively. The estimated 5-year overall and disease-free survivals were 37% and 33%, respectively. The 5-year local control rate was 59% with an estimated 5-year metastases-free survival of 36%.[80] Kresl and colleagues[81] described the Mayo clinic experience comprising 21 patients (12 who underwent R0 resection) who were treated with adjuvant 5-fluorouracil and radiation therapy. With a median follow-up of 5 years (range, 2.6–11 years), 5-year survival for the entire cohort was 33%. Median survival of the entire cohort was 2.6

years. The overall local control rate for the entire cohort at 1, 3, and 5 years was 90%, 73%, and 73%, respectively.[81]

A phase III randomized controlled trial compared adjuvant mitomycin C and 5-fluorouracil for GBCa.[82] A total of 69 patients with GBCa were treated compared with 43 observed after surgery. The 5-year overall survival rate was significantly better in the treated group (26%) compared with the control group (14.4%) ($P = .0367$). There was no difference in 5-year overall survival, however, among patients who received a curative resection (46.4% versus 30.9%; $P = .16$). The 5-year disease-free survival rate was 20.3% versus 11.6% among control patients ($P = .0210$). On multivariate analysis, postoperative adjuvant chemotherapy tended to reduce both the risk of death (HR = 0.654; $P = .0825$) and the risk of disease recurrence (HR = 0.626; $P = .0589$), although these reductions were not statistically significant. When the same analytic procedures were performed on patients without hepatic metastasis or peritoneal dissemination, postoperative adjuvant chemotherapy reduced the risk of death (HR = 0.551; $P = .0284$) and the risk of disease recurrence (HR = 0.569; $P = .0497$).[82]

SUMMARY

Aggressive tumor biology, high frequency of advanced disease at initial presentation, and the multitude of mechanisms of disease spread make the surgical management of GBCa challenging. The rarity of GBCa coupled with the prevalence of benign gallbladder disease mean that most patients undergo initial procedures that violate tumor planes, complicating attempts at future oncologic resection. Indeed, most cases of GBCa are discovered incidentally after cholecystectomy for benign disease. Although US may identify suspicious lesions preoperatively, CT or MRI are necessary to confirm the presence of tumors and to define resectability. There is limited role for PET in GBCa. Fortunately, a previous laparoscopic or open cholecystectomy does not alter survival after definitive surgical extirpation. Although sufficient for T1 disease, the high frequency of positive margins, regional lymph node disease, and vascular invasion make a simple cholecystectomy an unsatisfactory option for T2 disease or greater. Extended cholecystectomy (either as a primary procedure or in staged fashion after initial simple cholecystectomy) is the preferred for thicker tumors or regional nodal disease. Extended hepatectomy may also be an option in the setting of previous cholecystectomy where it is difficult to distinguish inflammatory scar tissue from tumor along the cystic plate. Although common bile duct resection may be useful in achieving margin-negative resection in cases where the cystic duct margin is involved with tumor, there is a lack of evidence showing survival benefit. Large retrospective and underpowered prospective studies have suggested benefit to adjuvant chemotherapy or radiotherapy; however, these results need to be confirmed with large prospective randomized trials.

REFERENCES

1. Miller G, Jarnagin WR. Gallbladder carcinoma. Eur J Surg Oncol 2008;34:306–12.
2. Fong Y, Jarnagin W, Blumgart LH. Gallbladder cancer: comparison of patients presenting initially for definitive operation with those presenting after prior noncurative intervention. Ann Surg 2000;232:557–69.
3. Cubertafond P, Gainant A, Cucchiaro G. Surgical treatment of 724 carcinomas of the gallbladder: results of the French Surgical Association survey. Ann Surg 1994; 219:275–80.

4. Benoist S, Panis Y, Fagniez PL, et al. Long-term results after curative resection for carcinoma of the gallbladder. Am J Surg 1998;175:118–22.
5. Gourgiotis S, Kocher HM, Solaini L, et al. Gallbladder cancer. Am J Surg 2008; 196:252–64.
6. Lazcano-Ponce EC, Miquel JF, Munoz N, et al. Epidemiology and molecular pathology of gallbladder cancer. CA Cancer J Clin 2001;51:349–64.
7. Donohoe JH, Nagorney DM, Grant CS, et al. Carcinoma of the gallbladder: does radical resection improve outcome? Arch Surg 1990;125:237–41.
8. Wistuba II, Gazdar AF. Gallbladder cancer: lessons from a rare tumor. Nat Rev Cancer 2004;4:695–706.
9. Barakat J, Dunkelberg JC, Ma TY. Changing patterns of gallbladder carcinoma in New Mexico. Cancer 2006;106:434–40.
10. Matsuda T, Marugame T. International comparisons of cumulative risk of gall-bladder cancer and other biliary tract cancer. From Cancer Incidence In Five Continents Vol. VIII. Jpn J Clin Oncol 2007;37:74–5.
11. Riandi G, Franceschi S, La Vecchia C. Gallbladder cancer worldwide: geograph-ical distribution and risk factors. Int J Cancer 2006;118:1591–602.
12. Kiran RP, Pokala N, Dudrick SJ. Incidence pattern and survival for gallbladder cancer over three decades: an analysis of 10301 patients. Ann Surg Oncol 2007;14:827–32.
13. Tazuma S, Kajiyama G. Carcinogenesis of malignant lesions of the gall bladder. Langenbecks Arch Surg 2001;386:224–9.
14. Csendes A, Becerra M, Rojas J, et al. Number and size of stones in patients with asymptomatic and symptomatic gallstones and gallbladder carcinoma: a prospective study of 592 cases. J Gastrointest Surg 2000;4:481–5.
15. Roa I, Ibacache G, Roa J, et al. Gallstones and gallbladder cancer-volume and weight of gallstones are associated with gallbladder cancer: a case-control study. J Surg Oncol 2006;93:624–8.
16. Chow WH, Johansen C, Grindley G, et al. Gallstones, cholecystectomy and risk of cancers of the liver, biliary tract and pancreas. Br J Cancer 1999;79:640–4.
17. Zatonski WA, Lowenfels AB, Boyle P, et al. Epidemiologic aspects of gallbladder cancer: a case-control study of the SEARCH Program of the International Agency for Research on Cancer. J Natl Cancer Inst 1997;89:1132–8.
18. Okamoto M, Okamoto H, Kitahara F, et al. Ultrasonographic evidence of associ-ation of polyps and stones with gallbladder cancer. Am J Gastroenterol 1999;94: 446–50.
19. Kimura W, Shimada H, Kuroda A, et al. Carcinoma of the gallbladder and extra-hepatic bile duct in autopsy cases of the aged, with special reference to its rela-tionship to gallstones. Am J Gastroenterol 1989;84:386–90.
20. Nervi F, Duarte I, Gómez G, et al. Frequency of gallbladder cancer in Chile, a high-risk area. Int J Cancer 1988;41:657–60.
21. Maringhini A, Moreau JA, Melton LJ III, et al. Gallstones, gallbladder cancer, and other gastrointestinal malignancies: an epidemiologic study in Rochester, Minne-sota. Ann Intern Med 1987;107:30–5.
22. Ishiguro S, Inoue M, Kurahashi N, et al. Risk factors of biliary tract cancer in a large-scale population based cohort study in Japan (JPHC study); with special focus on cholelithiasis, body mass index, and their effect modification. Cancer Causes Control 2008;19:33–41.
23. Hsing AW, Bai Y, Andreotii G, et al. Family history of gallstones and the risk of biliary tract cancer and gallstones: a population-based study in Shanghai, China. Int J Cancer 2007;121:832–8.

24. Yamagiwa H. Mucosal dysplasia of gallbladder: isolated and adjacent lesions to carcinoma. Jpn J Cancer Res 1989;80:238–43.
25. Oikarinen H. Diagnostic imaging of carcinomas of the gallbladder and the bile ducts. Acta Radiol 2006;4:345–58.
26. Rodriguez-Fernandez A, Gomez-Rio M, Medina-Benitez A. Application of modern imaging methods in diagnosis of gallbladder cancer. J Surg Oncol 2006;93: 650–64.
27. Pandey M, Sood BP, Shukla RC, et al. Carcinoma of the gallbladder: role of sonography in diagnosis and staging. J Clin Ultrasound 2000;28:227–32.
28. Grand D, Horton KM, Fishman EK. CT of the gallbladder: spectrum of disease. AJR Am J Roentgenol 2004;183:163–70.
29. Kim SJ, Lee JM, Lee JY, et al. Accuracy of preoperative T-staging of gallbladder carcinoma using MDCT. AJR Am J Roentgenol 2008;190:74–80.
30. Yoshimitsu K, Honda H, Shinozaki K, et al. Helical CT of the local spread of carcinoma of the gallbladder: evaluation according to the TNM system in patients who underwent surgical resection. AJR Am J Roentgenol 2002;179:423–8.
31. Kalra N, Suri S, Gupta R, et al. MDCT in the staging of gallbladder carcinoma. AJR Am J Roentgenol 2006;186:758–62.
32. Rao ND, Gulati MP, Paul SB, et al. Three-dimensional helical computed tomography cholangiography with minimum intensity projection in gallbladder carcinoma patients with obstructive jaundice: comparison with magnetic resonance cholangiography and percutaneous transhepatic cholangiography. J Gastroenterol Hepatol 2005;20:304–8.
33. Corvera CU, Blumgart LH, Akhurst T, et al. ^{18}F-fluorodeoxyglucose positron emission tomography influences management decisions in patients with biliary cancer. J Am Coll Surg 2008;206:57–65.
34. Petrowsky H, Wildbrett P, Husarik DB, et al. Impact of integrated positron emission tomography and computed tomography on staging and management of gallbladder cancer and cholangiocarcinoma. J Hepatol 2006;45:43–50.
35. Anderson CD, Rice MH, Pinson CW, et al. Fluorodeoxyglucose PET imaging in the evaluation of gallbladder carcinoma and cholangiocarcinoma. J Gastrointest Surg 2004;8:90–7.
36. Elsayes KM, Oliveira EP, Narra VR, et al. Magnetic resonance imaging of the gallbladder: spectrum of abnormalities. Acta Radiol 2007;48:476–82.
37. Kim JH, Kim TK, Eun HW, et al. Preoperative evaluation of gallbladder carcinoma: efficacy of combined use of MR imaging, MR cholangiography, and contrast-enhanced dual-phase three-dimensional MR angiography. J Magn Reson Imaging 2002;16:676–84.
38. American Joint Committee on Cancer. Gallbladder cancer. In: Greene FL, Page DL, editors. AJCC cancer staging manual. 6th edition. New York: Springer-Verlag; 2002. p. 139–42.
39. Fong Y, Wagman L, Gonen M, et al. Evidence-based gallbladder cancer staging. Ann Surg 2006;543:737–74.
40. Darmas B, Mahmud S, Abbas A, et al. Is there any justification for the routine histological examination of straightforward cholecystectomy specimens? Ann R Coll Surg Engl 2007;89:238–41.
41. Kwon A, Imamura A, Kitade H, et al. Unsuspected gallbladder cancer diagnosed during or after laparoscopic cholecystectomy. J Surg Oncol 2008;97:241–5.
42. Frauenschuh D, Greim R, Kraas E. How to proceed in patients with carcinoma detected after laparoscopic cholecystectomy. Langenbecks Arch Surg 2000;385: 495–500.

43. Foster JM, Hoshi H, Chu Q, et al. Radical re-resection is indicated for all T2 and T3 gallbladder and results in the same survival as primarily resected gallbladder cancers. Presented at the American Society of Clinical Oncology Gastrointestinal Cancers Symposium, January 27–29, 2005. Hollywood, CA. Abstr 140.
44. Taner CB, Nagorney DM, Donohue JH. Surgical treatment of gallbladder cancer. J Gastrointest Surg 2004;8:83–9.
45. Pawlik TM, Gleisner AL, Vigano L, et al. Incidence of finding residual disease for incidental gallbladder carcinoma: implications for re-resection. J Gastrointest Surg 2007;11:1478–87.
46. Yoshida T, Matsumoto T, Sasaki A, et al. Laparoscopic cholecystectomy in the treatment of patients with gallbladder cancer. J Am Coll Surg 2000;191:158–63.
47. Whalen GF, Bird I, Tanski W, et al. Laparoscopic cholecystectomy does not demonstrably decrease survival of patients with serendipitously treated gall-bladder cancer. J Am Coll Surg 2001;192:189–95.
48. Chan KM, Yeh TS, Jan YY, et al. Laparoscopic cholecystectomy for early gall-bladder carcinoma: long-term outcome in comparison with conventional open cholecystectomy. Surg Endosc 2006;20:1867–71.
49. Aretxabala XA, Roa IS, Mora JP, et al. Laparoscopic cholecystectomy: its effect on the prognosis of patients with gallbladder cancer. World J Surg 2004;28:544–7.
50. Sarli L, Contini S, Sansebastiano G, et al. Does laparoscopic cholecystectomy worsen the prognosis of unsuspected gallbladder cancer? Arch Surg 2000; 135:1340–4.
51. Toyonaga T, Chijiiwa K, Nakano K, et al. Completion radical surgery after chole-cystectomy for accidentally undiagnosed gallbladder carcinoma. World J Surg 2003;27:266–71.
52. Ito H, Matros E, Brooks DC, et al. Treatment outcomes associated with surgery for gallbladder cancer: a 20-year experience. J Gastrointest Surg 2004;8:183–90.
53. Ruckert JC, Ruckert RI, Gellert K, et al. Surgery for carcinoma of the gallbladder. Hepatogastroenterology 1996;43:527–33.
54. Behari A, Sikora SS, Wagholikar GD, et al. Longterm survival after extended resections in patients with gallbladder cancer. J Am Coll Surg 2003;196:82–8.
55. Shirai Y, Yoshida K, Tsukada K, et al. Radical surgery for gallbladder carcinoma: long-term results. Ann Surg 1992;216:565–8.
56. North JH, Pack MS, Hong C, et al. Prognostic factors for adenocarcinoma of the gallbladder: an analysis of 162 cases. Am Surg 1998;64:437–40.
57. Todoroki T, Kawamoto T, Takahashi H, et al. Treatment of gallbladder cancer by radical resection. Br J Surg 1999;86:622–7.
58. Kayahara M, Nagakawa T. Recent trends of gallbladder cancer in Japan: an anal-ysis of 4770 patients. Cancer 2007;110:572–80.
59. Schauer RJ, Meyer G, Baretton G, et al. Prognostic factors and long-term results after surgery for gallbladder carcinoma: a retrospective study of 127 patients. Langenbecks Arch Surg 2001;386:110–7.
60. Chan SY, Poon RTP, Lo CM, et al. Management of carcinoma of the gallbladder: a single institution experience in 16 years. J Surg Oncol 2008;97:156–64.
61. Balachandran P, Agarwal S, Krishnani N, et al. Predictors of long-term survival in patients with gallbladder cancer. J Gastrointest Surg 2006;10:848–54.
62. Kokudo N, Makuuchi M, Natori T, et al. Strategies for surgical treatment for gall-bladder carcinoma based on information available before resection. Arch Surg 2003;138:741–50.
63. Puhalla H, Wild T, Bareck E, et al. Long-term follow-up of surgically treated gall-bladder cancer patients. Eur J Surg Oncol 2002;28:857–63.

64. Yildirim E, Celen O, Gulben K, et al. The surgical management of incidental gall-bladder carcinoma. Eur J Surg Oncol 2005;31:45–52.
65. Kohya N, Miyazaki K. Hepatectomy of segment 4a and 5 combined with extra-hepatic bile duct resection for T2 and T3 gallbladder carcinoma. J Surg Oncol 2008;97:498–502.
66. Yagi H, Shimazu M, Kawachi S, et al. Retrospective analysis of outcome in 63 gallbladder carcinoma patients after radical resection. J Hepatobiliary Pancreat Surg 2006;13:530–6.
67. Kai M, Chijiiwa K, Ohuchida J, et al. A curative resection improves the postoper-ative survival rate even in patients with advanced gallbladder carcinoma. J Gas-trointest Surg 2007;11:1025–32.
68. Kang CM, Lee WJ, Choi GH, et al. Does clinical R0 have validity in the choice of simple cholecystectomy for gallbladder carcinoma? J Gastrointest Surg 2007;11: 1309–16.
69. Goetze TO, Paolucci V. Benefits of reoperation of T2 and more advanced inci-dental gallbladder carcinoma. Ann Surg 2008;247:104–8.
70. Ouchi K, Mikuni J, Kakugawa Y. Laparoscopic cholecystectomy for gallbladder carcinoma: results of a Japanese survey of 498 patients. J Hepatobiliary Pan-creat Surg 2002;9:256–60.
71. Jensen EH, Abraham A, Habermann EB, et al. Cholecystectomy alone versus radical resection for early-stage gallbladder cancer. Presented at the 2008 Amer-ican Society of Clinical Oncology Gastrointestinal Cancers Symposium, January 25–27, 2008. Orlando, FL. Abstr 195.
72. Foster JM, Hoshi H, Gibbs JF, et al. Gallbladder cancer: defining the indications for primary radical resection and radical re-resection. Ann Surg Oncol 2007;14: 833–40.
73. Coburn NG, Cleary SP, Tan JCC, et al. Surgery for gallbladder cancer: a popula-tion-based analysis. J Am Coll Surg 2008;207:371–82.
74. Wright BE, Lee CC, Iddings DM, et al. Management of T2 gallbladder cancer: are practice patterns consistent with national recommendations? Am J Surg 2007; 194:820–6.
75. Sakamoto Y, Kosuge T, Shimada K, et al. Clinical significance of extrahepatic bile duct resection for advanced gallbladder cancer. J Surg Oncol 2006;94:298–306.
76. Reddy SK, Marroquin CE, Kuo PC, et al. Extended hepatic resection for gall-bladder cancer. Am J Surg 2007;194:355–61.
77. Wang SJ, Fuller D, Kim JS, et al. Prediction model for estimating the survival benefit of adjuvant radiotherapy for gallbladder cancer. J Clin Oncol 2008;26:2112–7.
78. Todoroki T, Kawamoto T, Otsuka M. Benefits of combining radiotherapy with aggressive resection for stage IV gallbladder cancer. Hepatogastroenterology 1999;46:1585–91.
79. Atiq M, Safa MM, Komrokji RS, et al. Improvement in survival in VA patients with gallbladder cancer given chemotherapy. Presented at the 2006 American Society of Clinical Oncology Annual Meeting, June 2–6, 2006. Atlanta GA. Abstr 4132.
80. Czito BG, Hurwitz HI, Clough RW, et al. Adjuvant external-beam radiotherapy with concurrent chemotherapy after resection of primary gallbladder carcinoma: a 23-year experience. Int J Radiat Oncol Biol Phys 2005;62:1030–4.
81. Kresl JJ, Schild SE, Henning GT, et al. Adjuvant external beam radiation therapy with concurrent chemotherapy in the management of gallbladder carcinoma. Int J Radiat Oncol Biol Phys 2002;52:167–75.
82. Takada T, Amano H, Yasuda H. Is postoperative adjuvant chemotherapy useful for gallbladder carcinoma? Cancer 2002;95:1685–95.

Transplantation for Cholangiocarcinoma: When and for Whom?

David J. Rea, MD[a], Charles B. Rosen, MD[a],*, David M. Nagorney, MD[b], Julie K. Heimbach, MD[a], Gregory J. Gores, MD[c]

KEYWORDS

- Cholangiocarcinoma • Liver transplantation • Neoadjuvant
- Chemotherapy • Radiation • Outcomes

Cholangiocarcinoma (CCA) is a rare malignancy arising from the cholangiocytes of the intrahepatic and extrahepatic bile ducts and accounts for approximately 5000 new cases of cancer annually in the United States.[1] A recent overview from the Surveillance Epidemiology and End Results database demonstrated that the incidence of intrahepatic CCA (which includes hilar CCA) has increased from 0.32 per 100,000 (1975–1979) to 0.85 per 100,000 (1995–1999).[2] Conversely, the incidence of extrahepatic CCA seems to have decreased over the same time period.[3]

The treatment of hilar CCA with only bile duct resection provided dismal results until Launois and coworkers[4] in 1979 reported a large series of patients treated with combined bile duct and hepatic resection. Since that time, the surgical standard of care has evolved to include extrahepatic bile duct resection, regional lymphadenectomy, and hepatectomy with bilioenteric continuity restored by hepaticojejunostomy.[5,6] Unfortunately, only 20% to 30% of patients are candidates for resection, with the remaining patients having unresectable or metastatic disease. The difficulty with resection is that the tumor lies in close proximity to the portal vein and hepatic artery bifurcations, and vascular encasement is common. Hepatic artery and portal venous reconstruction are occasionally performed to enable resection of tumor involving the vasculature to the remnant liver. The surgical treatment of CCA arising in patients with primary sclerosing cholangitis (PSC) has also been disappointing.[7,8] These tumors often are multicentric and unresectable, either because of the local extent of disease or underlying liver disease (eg, PSC).

[a] Division of Transplantation Surgery, Mayo Clinic College of Medicine, 200 First Street SW, Rochester, MN 55905, USA
[b] Division of Gastrointestinal and General Surgery, Mayo Clinic College of Medicine, 200 First Street SW, Rochester, MN 55905, USA
[c] Division of Gastroenterology and Hepatology, Mayo Clinic College of Medicine, 200 First Street SW, Rochester, MN 55905, USA
* Corresponding author.
E-mail address: rosen.charles@mayo.edu (C.B. Rosen).

Surg Oncol Clin N Am 18 (2009) 325–337
doi:10.1016/j.soc.2008.12.008   surgonc.theclinics.com
1055-3207/08/$ – see front matter © 2009 Elsevier Inc. All rights reserved.

Many institutions now consider CCA a contraindication for liver transplantation. During the past 15 years, however, the authors' group has used a regimen of neoadjuvant radiation and chemotherapy followed by liver transplantation in selected patients with hilar CCA. This article describes the history of transplantation for CCA, the evolution of the current protocol, and the results of the authors' experience. Also discussed is prioritization for organ allocation in this unique group of patients and the future of transplantation in reference to more aggressive surgical approaches that are being undertaken.

BACKGROUND

At the dawn of liver transplantation, CCA seemed to be the ideal indication for the procedure. Liver transplantation would achieve wide tumor-free margins along the biliary tree; address vascular and hepatic parenchymal invasion; and effectively treat underlying liver disease (eg, PSC). Despite this sound theoretical argument in favor of liver transplantation for CCA, early results did not bear this out.

Several early studies focusing on liver transplantation for PSC have touched on outcomes with incidentally discovered CCA. A 12-year review of liver transplantation for PSC from the University of California Los Angeles group identified 10 patients transplanted for incidental CCA and 4 with known CCA.[9] Although the survival in patients with incidental CCA was similar to PSC patients without CCA (1-, 2-, and 5-year survivals of 90%, 88%, 87%), survival for the patients with known CCA was significantly lower (1-, 2-, and 5-year survival of 33%, 33%, 0%; $P<.0001$ for the comparison). In contrast, data from the Mayo Clinic and the University of Pittsburgh demonstrated poor survival for PSC patients with incidental CCA. Five-year survival in patients with PSC and incidental CCA was 47% compared with 75% in patients with PSC alone ($P = .02$).[10]

A Canadian study by Gahli and colleagues[11] confirmed the poor outcome associated with incidental CCA. They reviewed the Canadian experience from 1996 through June 2003 with undetected CCA that was discovered in the explant after successful liver transplantation. Eighty percent (8 of 10) of these tumors arose in patients with PSC and 60% of tumors were extrahepatic. Most of these incidental tumors were less than 1 cm, none had any perihepatic lymph node involvement, and 90% had well or moderately differentiated histology. Despite these favorable characteristics, 3-year survival was only 30%. Eighty percent of patients experienced tumor recurrence at a median time of 26 months. The study was too small to examine any prognostic variables.

The Cincinnati Tumor Registry reported patients transplanted for the diagnosis of CCA from 1968 to 1997.[12] One year, 3-year, and 5-year survivals were 72%, 48%, and 23%, respectively. The recurrence rate was 51%, with a median time to recurrence of 9.7 months. The median survival after recurrence was only 2 months. Negative prognostic variables were tumor metastases to the regional lymph nodes and tumor extension to adjacent local structures (eg, duodenum and portal vein). Interestingly, incidentally detected CCA had survival equivalent to tumors diagnosed before transplantation. This study is limited, however, in that it does not distinguish between patients with intrahepatic and hilar CCA, tumors that have distinctly different biologic behaviors.

A recent report from a consortium of Spanish transplant centers on the results for liver transplantation for CCA had similar results.[13] They reviewed 59 patients who underwent liver transplantation for CCA (39 hilar and 23 peripheral [eg, intrahepatic]) from 1988 to 2001. The 1-, 3-, and 5-year survival for hilar CCA was 82%, 53%, and 30% compared with 77%, 65%, and 42% for intrahepatic CCA. The recurrence rates were 53% and 35% in the two groups, and tumor recurrence was also the main cause of death in both groups. The poor prognostic variables for hilar CCA included the presence of vascular invasion and tumor stage III or greater. Although the survival in these patients is less than that for liver transplantation performed for other indications, the 30% to 42% 5-year survival seen in these transplant patients who were otherwise not candidates for standard surgical therapy is far better than that achieved with palliative radiation therapy alone.

Becker and colleagues[14] reviewed the United Network for Organ Sharing (UNOS) database examining the results of liver transplantation for CCA. Two-hundred eighty patients underwent liver transplant from 1987 to 2005 with a diagnosis of CCA. Overall 1-year and 5-year survival were 74% and 38%, respectively. Fifty-five (48%) of 114 patient deaths were caused by locally recurrent or metastatic CCA. The poor prognostic variables noted in this study included pretransplant location (ICU and hospital versus home); serum creatinine greater than or equal to 2 mg/dL; and serum bilirubin greater than or equal to 2 mg/dL. This study noted that there was no significant difference in survival between patients transplanted early in the experience (before 1994, when oncologic information was not routinely collected) compared with later (1995 and later). There was a significant survival difference, however, in patients transplanted after 1995 who had known CCA versus incidentally discovered CCA (5-year survivals of 68% and 20%, respectively [$P<.001$]). Presumably, this series included a number of patients from the authors' own institution treated with the protocol described later, which in part explains the improved survival in patients with known disease.

NEOADJUVANT THERAPY

Adjuvant radiation therapy for CCA has limited value after surgical resection, but early results using neoadjuvant chemoradiation in patients who underwent resection were promising.[15] McMasters and colleagues[16] reported on 40 patients who underwent resection for CCA; 18 (45%) had postoperative chemoradiation and 9 (23%) had preoperative chemoradiation. There were no differences in overall survival between the patients treated with preoperative chemoradiation, postoperative chemoradiation, or resection alone. The preoperative chemoradiation group, however, had tumor-free margins in 100% of specimens ($P<.0001$ versus other groups), and three patients had complete pathologic responses. The neoadjuvant chemoradiation group only had minor postoperative complications.

Early indications that radiation and chemotherapy may be useful in a neoadjuvant setting also came from experience at Thomas Jefferson University and the authors' own institution.[17,18] In the Mayo Clinic series, 24 patients with extrahepatic CCA were treated with external beam radiotherapy (median dose, 50.4 Gy) followed by transcatheter brachytherapy by endoscopic retrograde cholangiopancreatography or percutaneous transhepatically placed wires (median dose at 1 cm radius was 20 Gy). Nine patients received concomitant 5-fluorouracil during treatment. Five patients had grade 1 tumor, nine had grade 2, six had grade 3, and one had grade 4 disease. Median survival was 12.8 months (range, 7.5 months–9 years). The overall 5-year survival rate was 14.1%, with three patients surviving more than 5 years after therapy. One patient survived without relapse 10 years from diagnosis and 5 years after liver transplantation for liver failure. There seemed to be a trend toward improved survival with the addition of 5-fluorouracil chemotherapy. Although no patients underwent resection in this cohort, the fact that 14% of patients with advanced CCA could survive 5 years or more with radiation therapy alone suggested that patients may derive some benefit by slowing the growth of the CCA.

The use of neoadjuvant radiation therapy before liver transplantation was pioneered at the University of Nebraska. The University of Nebraska most recently reported their experience with 17 patients considered for liver transplantation for CCA.[19] Their protocol used only intrabiliary brachytherapy delivered through iridium-192 wires, to a total dose of 6000 cGy. The patients then received daily intravenous 5-flurouracil until the time of transplantation. At the time of transplantation an exploratory laparotomy was performed with pathologic examination of regional lymph nodes. If the tumor had extrahepatic spread or lymph node involvement, the liver was allocated to an alternate recipient. One of the 17 patients had a fatal septic complication before transplantation and 5 of 17 had tumor progression precluding transplantation (35% dropout rate). Of the 11 patients undergoing liver transplantation, six patients died (three within 12 weeks of surgery because of hemorrhage or infection) and the overall median survival was 25 months. Two patients (18%) had documented recurrences. Despite the significant morbidity and mortality in their study, the overall 5-year survival rate was 30%. The Nebraska group was encouraged by their results and stated that improved patient selection, improved staging, and prevention and treatment of infectious complications would further improve the results.

Given the past failure of liver transplantation alone for CCA and the apparent benefits of neoadjuvant radiation and chemotherapy, a collaborative group of surgeons, gastroenterologists, hepatologists, medical oncologists, and radiation oncologists at the Mayo Clinic developed a protocol for neoadjuvant chemoradiotherapy followed by liver transplantation for patients with CCA in 1993. The protocol is based on rigorous patient selection, bimodal neoadjuvant radiation with concomitant chemotherapy, operative staging of patients before committing to transplantation, and subsequent liver transplantation using either deceased or living donors. The general outline of the approach is shown in **Fig. 1**.

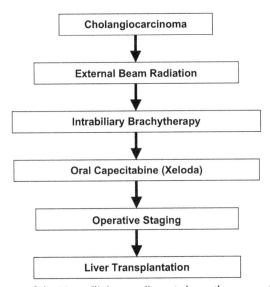

Fig. 1. General schema of the Mayo Clinic neoadjuvant chemotherapy and liver transplantation protocol for CCA. Please see the text for details.

PATIENT SELECTION

The inclusion criteria for patients with CCA are shown in **Box 1**. The protocol involves careful selection of patients with early stage CCA either deemed locally unresectable by an experienced hepatobiliary surgeon or arising in the setting of underlying PSC. The original criteria required that the hilar CCA not extend lower than the cystic duct, but it was subsequently found that microscopic CCA arising in PSC located in the common bile duct is amenable to transplantation when combined with pancreato-duodenectomy. Currently, patients are only eligible for the protocol if there is no mass lesion below the level of the cystic duct. If there is microscopic disease suspected below this level, patients are enrolled with the intent of performing a pancreaticoduo-denectomy at the time of the liver transplantation, assuming that operative staging is otherwise negative.

Vascular encasement of the hilar vessels is not a contraindication to transplantation. The upper limit of tumor size is 3 cm when a mass is visible on cross-sectional imaging studies, and there must be no evidence for intrahepatic or extrahepatic metastases by any imaging modality (chest CT, abdominal CT, abdominal MRI, ultrasonography, or bone scan). The protocol specifically excludes patients with intrahepatic CCA or gall-bladder involvement. Surgical intervention and percutaneous biopsy are avoided before protocol enrollment to minimize perioperative complications and tumor recur-rence. Patients who have had transperitoneal biopsy or violation of the bile duct during a prior attempt at surgical resection are disqualified because peritoneal seeding has been encountered in these patients. Candidates must have received no other treat-ment before neoadjuvant therapy, and have no active infections or medical conditions that preclude neoadjuvant therapy or liver transplantation.

The authors have recently reported on their experience with endoscopic ultrasound as a selection tool in patients with CCA treated with the protocol.[20] Since 2002, they have used endoscopic ultrasound-guided regional lymph node aspiration routinely in

---

Box 1
Diagnostic criteria for cholangiocarcinoma in the Mayo protocol

Definitive diagnostic criteria

- Biopsy (transluminal) positive for cancer
- Positive or suspicious cytology on brush cytology
- Stricture, and FISH polysomy
- Mass lesion on cross-sectional imaging
- Malignant-appearing stricture and CA-19.9 >100 U/mL or FISH polysomy

Indeterminate diagnostic criteria

- FISH trisomy (7 or 3)
- Dysplasia
- DIA >1.8 in isolation (FISH negative, routine cytology negative)
- FISH polysomy in absence of malignant-appearing stricture
- Malignant-appearing stricture in absence of mass lesion, positive cytology, biopsy, elevated CA-19.9, or FISH polysomy

Abbreviations: CA-19.9, Carcinoembryonic antigen 19.9; DIA, Digital image analysis; FISH, Fluo-rescence in-situ hybridization.

all patients before beginning neoadjuvant therapy. Forty-seven patients had a total of 70 lymph nodes sampled, with nine (11%) malignant lymph nodes identified in eight (17%) separate patients. There were no morphologic features (eg, size, echogenicity, borders) of the lymph nodes that predicted metastases. All identified lymph nodes visualized during the procedure were routinely sampled. The identification of lymph node metastases obviated the need for exploratory laparotomy and disqualified the patients from subsequent liver transplantation. Since the time routine endoscopic ultrasound-guided regional lymph node aspiration began, 13 other patients were disqualified from the protocol for other reasons (distant metastases, prior surgery, and so forth). Twenty-two patients underwent exploratory laparotomy and 20 (91%) were confirmed to be lymph node negative. With the introduction of routine endoscopic ultrasound in the protocol, the percentage of patients with a positive staging laparotomy (described later) has decreased from 30% to 15%.

MAYO PROTOCOL
Neoadjuvant Therapy

Neoadjuvant therapy (4000–4500 cGy) is administered by external beam radiation, followed by transcatheter radiation (2000–3000 cGy) with iridium-192 wires. These wires are placed by endoscopic retrograde cholangiography or percutaneous transhepatic cholangiography. Infusional 5-flurouracil is given during the radiation treatment and followed by oral capecitabine (Xeloda) after the radiation therapy until the day of transplantation.

Staging Operation

Before transplantation, patients undergo a staging abdominal exploration, a procedure that is crucial in the overall management of these patients. The staging operation involves a thorough abdominal exploration. At least one lymph node along the proper hepatic artery and another along the common bile duct are excised even if the regional nodes seem normal. The liver is carefully palpated for evidence of intrahepatic metastases that may have gone undetected by preoperative imaging studies. The caudate is examined to determine if a caval-sparing hepatectomy is possible (necessary for living donor liver transplantation). Regional lymph node metastases, peritoneal metastases, or locally extensive disease preclude transplantation. Selected patients without any prior upper abdominal operations (including laparoscopic cholecystectomy) have more recently been staged with a hand-assisted laparoscopic approach, which seems to speed patient recovery compared with an open approach.

In patients who have opted to have a living donor liver transplant, the staging operation is performed a day or two before the living donor transplant. In patients without living donors, the staging operation is usually done as the time nears for transplantation. Patients are registered on the deceased donor transplant waiting list with an appealed model for end-stage liver disease (MELD) score per a cooperative agreement with the other liver transplant programs in UNOS Region 7.

Liver Transplantation

The liver transplant operation is performed through a standard bilateral subcostal incision with a superior extension in the midline. Hilar dissection is avoided to prevent violation of the tumor and the portal vein is divided as low as possible, close to the pancreas. In most cases a caval-sparing hepatectomy can be performed. If there is concern for tumor extension into the caudate (found at staging or at the time of hepatectomy) the retrohepatic cava is excised and the new liver implanted with the caval interposition technique. The bile duct is transected at the level of the pancreas and the margin is submitted for frozen section examination. If there is microscopic tumor involvement, a concomitant pancreaticoduodenectomy is also performed (see later). In deceased donor transplants arterial inflow is reconstructed with a donor iliac artery graft from the infrarenal aorta. This approach was tried in the early living donor transplant experience but had problems with arterial thrombosis. Using the native common hepatic artery, despite its exposure to radiation during the neoadjuvant therapy, is now favored. Use of the native hepatic artery results in a 20% late stenosis rate. The native portal vein is used in deceased donor transplants, whereas in living donor liver transplants a portal vein interposition graft is routinely constructed using a small segment of blood group–compatible deceased donor iliac vein. Bilioenteric continuity is restored with a standard Roux-en-Y hepaticojejunostomy or choledochojejunostomy. The CCA patients receive the standard immunosuppression regimen of steroids, followed by tacrolimus (Prograf), and mycophenolate mofetil (CellCept). Baring any acute cellular rejection, patients are maintained on tacrolimus monotherapy after 4 months.

Long-term follow-up includes abdominal and chest CT and CA-19.9 levels at 4 months and every year after transplantation. Portal and arterial flow is also routinely followed by both CT and ultrasound to detect late vascular complications.

RESULTS

The first published results of the protocol were encouraging.[21] Twenty-five patients were evaluated for the protocol and six were deemed unacceptable candidates for the neoadjuvant chemoradiotherapy because of metastases. Of the 19 remaining patients who underwent neoadjuvant therapy, a single patient died from overwhelming biliary sepsis. At staging laparotomy, 6 (33%) of the 18 patients had peritoneal metastases or regional lymph node involvement that precluded transplantation. Twelve patients underwent transplantation. Patient survival after transplantation was 100% with a median follow-up of 44 months. There was a single tumor recurrence at 40 months. This recurrence occurred in a patient with a stage IVa tumor discovered in the explant; all the remaining patients had stage I or II tumors. Graft survival was 91%, because one patient required retransplantation for hepatic artery thrombosis within 30 days of transplantation.

In 2004 the authors performed a retrospective comparison of their institutional experience using neoadjuvant chemoradiation combined with liver transplantation for patients with unresectable disease or underlying PSC to their experience with resection for patients with resectable disease.[22] The patients were treated over an 11-year period and were not randomized to therapy; patients deemed resectable were treated with major hepatectomy and extrahepatic bile duct resection, those who were unresectable or had underlying PSC were preferentially enrolled in the transplant protocol. Seventy-one patients were enrolled in the transplant protocol; 9 patients died or had disease progression before staging laparotomy, 14 patients had positive staging operations, and 10 patients were either awaiting staging or liver transplantation at the end of the study period. Thirty-eight patients were transplanted during the study period. During this same period, 54 patients were explored for resection. Fifty-two percent (28 patients) had findings precluding a curative resection, and 26 patients underwent hepatectomy. The two groups were significantly different in that the transplant group was younger (mean age, 48 years versus 63 years) and the transplant patients had a higher incidence of PSC and inflammatory bowel disease (58% and 31% in the transplant patients versus 8% and 8% in the resection patients). Patient survivals at 1, 3, and 5 years after liver transplantation were 92%, 82%, and

82% compared 82%, 48%, and 21% after resection (P = .022). In the de novo CCA group (without underlying PSC), the 1-, 3-, and 5-year survivals were 94%, 71%, and 71% in the transplant protocol group compared with 83%, 42%, and 18% in the resection group.

The cohorts are very different in terms of age and underlying disease, and these differences may have accounted for some of the survival differences between the groups. Thirty-day mortality was 12% in the resection group compared with 0% in the transplant group, indicating that the resected patients were probably less able to withstand complications after major surgery. Nevertheless, CCA patients with unresectable disease or damaged hepatic parenchyma had better survival than patients with resectable disease treated with standard resection.

The authors also identified prognostic factors for recurrence of CCA after transplantation.[23] Out of the 106 patients entered into the protocol by January 2006, 65 patients had successfully completed neoadjuvant therapy, underwent staging laparotomy, and had a successful liver transplant. With a mean follow-up of 32 months, 5-year actuarial survival in this group was 76%. Eleven patients (17%) had documented recurrence after transplantation. Variables that predicted tumor recurrence included age at the time of transplant; pretransplant CA-19.9 level greater than 100 U/mL; prior cholecystectomy; residual (viable) tumor grater than 2 cm in the explant; presence of a mass on pretransplant imaging; perineural tumor invasion; and advanced tumor grade. It was also noted that the recurrence rate was lower in patients who underwent liver transplantation closer in time to the staging operation.

Since 1993, the authors have performed 10 concomitant pancreaticoduodenectomies at the time of liver transplantation. All of these patients had underlying PSC; no patient with de novo CCA has required a Whipple operation. Seven patients had microscopically positive common bile duct margins noted at the time of transplant, which prompted the pancreaticoduodenectomy. Five patients are alive and disease-free (1–9 years after transplantation) and two patients died because of hepatic artery thrombosis within 3 months of transplantation. Two patients with PSC and prior biliary tract surgery had en bloc pancreaticoduodenectomy at the time of transplantation; both patients are alive and without recurrence 2 and 5 years after transplantation. One recent patient had tumor located in both the common hepatic duct and a known microscopic focus in the common bile duct. An en bloc pancreaticoduodenectomy was performed in this case, and the patient is well 2 months following transplantation. Overall, 15% of PSC patients have had positive distal bile duct margins.

As of September 2008, 167 patients have been entered into the protocol (**Fig. 2**). Twelve patients died or dropped out during the neoadjuvant chemoradiotherapy, 2

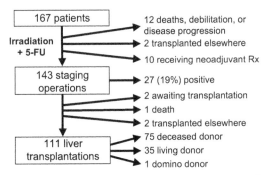

Fig. 2. Patient outcomes and current dispositions (as of September 2008) of the 167 patients enrolled in the Mayo Clinic liver transplantation protocol for CCA.

went on to transplantation elsewhere, and 10 patients were currently receiving neoadjuvant therapy. Of the 143 patients who underwent operative staging, 27 patients (19%) had findings precluding transplantation. Two patients are awaiting liver transplantation, one patient died while waiting for a liver, and two patients sought transplantation elsewhere. Of the 111 patients who underwent liver transplantation, 75 (67%) received deceased donor livers; 35 (32%) received living donor livers; and 1 (1%) received a domino liver (an explanted liver from a recipient with familial amyloidosis). Current 1-, 3-, and 5-year patient survivals after the start of therapy (N = 167) are 84%, 64%, and 56% (**Fig. 3**). Current 1-, 3-, and 5-year patient survivals after liver transplantation (N = 111) are 96%, 83%, and 72% (**Fig. 4**). There is no difference in survival between the patients receiving a deceased donor liver compared with a living donor liver. There have been 15 recurrences in the 111 liver transplant patients (14%), occurring at a mean of 25 months after transplantation (range, 7–64 months).

COMPLICATIONS

Infectious complications related to the treatment of CCA are very common before transplantation. Cholangitis is a frequent cause for hospital admission for patients with indwelling biliary stents to relieve malignant obstruction. Patients are at risk to develop intrahepatic abscesses caused by both neoadjuvant radiation-induced tumor necrosis and prolonged biliary obstruction in the setting of PSC. Gastritis, duodenitis, and poor gastric emptying are fairly common, and several patients have required operative intervention for duodenal ulceration with perforation or catastrophic bleeding. These problems can persist or develop after transplantation.

Patients treated with neoadjuvant therapy are at risk for long-term vascular complications after transplantation.[24] In a study of 68 patients, 21% developed arterial complications and 20% of patients developed portal venous complications, most commonly stenosis with or without thrombosis. The native common hepatic artery is avoided during deceased donor transplantation, but its use in living donor transplantation is associated with a 20% late stenosis-thrombosis rate. Late hepatic artery complications occurred more often in living donor recipients transplanted for CCA than patients with other diagnoses ($P = .047$). Late portal vein complications occurred more often in both whole organ and living donor recipients transplanted for CCA compared with control groups ($P = .01$ and $P = .009$). Hepatic venous complications are rare. Patient and graft survival are not different between CCA and control patients. Although liver transplantation after neoadjuvant therapy is associated with higher rates

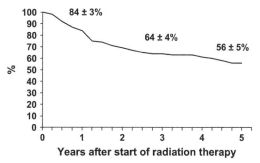

Fig. 3. The Kaplan-Meier survival curve for all patients (N = 167, see **Fig. 2**) treated under the protocol since 1993 from the start of radiation therapy (through September 2008).

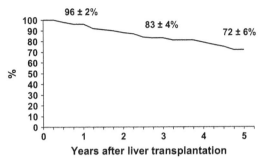

Fig. 4. The Kaplan-Meier survival curve for all patients (N = 111, see **Fig. 2**) who have undergone liver transplantation since 1993 (through September 2008).

of late arterial and portal venous complications, these complications have not adversely affected patient and graft survival.

ORGAN ALLOCATION

Prioritization for deceased donor liver allocation is highly controversial and was discussed in detail by an international group of transplant surgeons and physicians at the MELD Exception Study Group, Chicago, March 1–2, 2006.[25] The MELD Exception Study Group concluded that current data justify prioritization similar to that for hepatocellular carcinoma for patients enrolled in clinical trials provided that (1) transplant centers submit formal patient care protocols to the UNOS Liver and Intestinal Committee; (2) candidates satisfy accepted diagnostic criteria for CCA and be considered unresectable on the basis of technical considerations or underlying liver disease (eg, PSC); (3) tumor mass, when visible on cross-sectional imaging studies, be less than 3 cm in diameter; (4) imaging studies to assess patients for intrahepatic and extrahepatic metastases be repeated before interval score increases; (5) regional hepatic lymph node involvement and the peritoneal cavity be assessed by operative staging after completion of neoadjuvant therapy and before transplantation; and (6) transperitoneal aspiration or biopsy of the primary tumor be avoided because of the high risk of tumor seeding associated with these procedures.

UNRESOLVED ISSUES

The authors' institution continues to offer major hepatectomy and extrahepatic bile duct resection to patients who have resectable de novo hilar CCA. It is also clear, however, that liver transplantation for hilar CCA using the Mayo Protocol results in prolonged survival in a group of patients that are not candidates for conventional surgical therapy. These groups have been compared retrospectively and it was found that the liver transplantation patients had better survival than conventionally treated patients. The difference in survival may be attributable to efficacy of the aggressive neoadjuvant therapy; the more radical resection achieved by hepatectomy; patient selection (eg, operatively staged node-negative disease); or, more likely, a combination of these three factors.

One might consider administration of neoadjuvant therapy to patients with potentially resectable disease with a plan to proceed with resection rather than transplantation. Unfortunately, neoadjuvant therapy causes significant bile duct injury, which precludes biliary reconstruction after resection. Indeed, the major hepatic ducts show widespread necrosis and sclerosis in the explanted livers. Even if resection and biliary reconstruction were technically possible, the remaining liver is at high risk for liver failure to the long-term effects of radiation.

Liver transplantation achieves a more radical resection than is possible with conventional hepatic resection. Although the widespread hilar sclerosis and necrosis evident in the livers may hinder pathologic examination, the authors do find residual carcinoma in approximately half of the specimens (Rosen, unpublished data, 2009). Without liver transplantation, all of these patients with residual disease would likely succumb, either from tumor progression or liver failure caused by the radiation therapy.

The question then remains whether the liver transplantation protocol should be applied to cases of de novo CCA that are candidates for surgical resection. Would one achieve better survival and lower recurrence rates? The most objective way of answering this question is to conduct a randomized controlled trial comparing these two therapies. Such a trial requires randomization before neoadjuvant therapy or operative staging assessment of resectability. Patients need to understand that there is no opportunity for crossover between the treatment arms. Patients (from the transplant arm) who at the time of staging laparotomy are found to have lymph nodes metastases would not be able to undergo resection. Similarly, patients who at the time of resection are found to have unresectable disease would be poor candidates for liver transplantation because of significant risk of tumor dissemination from the exploration.

Several recent reports have demonstrated excellent results using vascular reconstruction in conjunction with extended hepatic resections.[26,27] The 5-year survival in these selected groups is approximately 65%. Neuhaus and colleagues[26] have also used liver transplantation and pancreaticoduodenectomy, although they did not use neoadjuvant radiation in their protocol. In these studies the transplant cohort had the highest rates of R0 resection (93%) but with a poorer overall 5-year survival (38%). Neuhaus and colleagues[26] reported excellent results with extended hepatectomy and portal vein reconstruction. Their patient survival compared favorably with the authors' transplant data. Neuhaus and colleagues[26] survival data, however, excludes patients who died in the perioperative period (between 0 and 60 days after the procedure). If the perioperative deaths were included in the analysis, the patient survival at 5 years would certainly be reduced. With better selection of these patients, the perioperative mortality could likely be reduced with an improvement in overall survival. Perhaps this group of patients is a more similar control group to compare with the patients entered into the liver transplant protocol because they are all unresectable by conventional techniques.

SUMMARY

The role of liver transplantation for treatment of CCA has undergone significant evolution during the last 15 years. Early results of liver transplantation alone were poor and CCA became an accepted contraindication. With rigorous patient selection, inclusion of neoadjuvant radiation therapy, operative staging to identify node-negative patients, and subsequent liver transplantation, the protocol has achieved excellent results. Currently, the authors have attained 72% 5-year survival for patients with unresectable CCA or CCA arising in the setting of PSC. These results exceed those of resection for patients with resectable disease. Neoadjuvant therapy does cause significant morbidity before and after transplantation, but does not preclude a successful outcome.

Liver transplantation with neoadjuvant chemoradiotherapy has secured a place in the treatment of selected patients with hilar CCA. In the future, as surgical techniques advance, new radiation modalities are introduced, and new chemotherapeutic agents are developed, the standard of care for CCA will change. The protocol also will change over time, incorporating these new advancements as they apply to the patients evaluated for this therapy. The results with neoadjuvant chemoradiotherapy and liver transplantation for patients with CCA exceed all reported results with resection. In the future application of this approach to patients with potentially resectable disease needs to be considered.

REFERENCES

1. de Groen PC, Gores GJ, LaRusso NF, et al. Biliary tract cancers. N Engl J Med 1999;341(18):1368–78.
2. Shaib YH, Davila JA, McGlynn K, et al. Rising incidence of intrahepatic cholangiocarcinoma in the United States: a true increase? J Hepatol 2004;40(3):472–7.
3. Shaib Y, El-Serag HB. The epidemiology of cholangiocarcinoma. Semin Liver Dis 2004;24(2):115–25.
4. Launois B, Campion JP, Brissot P, et al. Carcinoma of the hepatic hilus: surgical management and the case for resection. Ann Surg 1979;190(2):151–7.
5. Rea DJ, Munoz-Juarez M, Farnell MB, et al. Major hepatic resection for hilar cholangiocarcinoma: analysis of 46 patients. Arch Surg 2004;139(5):514–23 [discussion 523–5].
6. Hemming AW, Reed AI, Fujita S, et al. Surgical management of hilar cholangiocarcinoma. Ann Surg 2005;241(5):693–9 [discussion 699–702].
7. Rosen CB, Nagorney DM, Wiesner RH, et al. Cholangiocarcinoma complicating primary sclerosing cholangitis. Ann Surg 1991;213(1):21–5.
8. Rosen CB, Nagorney DM. Cholangiocarcinoma complicating primary sclerosing cholangitis. Semin Liver Dis 1991;11(1):26–30.
9. Goss JA, Shackleton CR, Farmer DG, et al. Orthotopic liver transplantation for primary sclerosing cholangitis: a 12-year single center experience. Ann Surg 1997;225(5):472–81 [discussion 481–3].
10. Abu-Elmagd KM, Malinchoc M, Dickson ER, et al. Efficacy of hepatic transplantation in patients with primary sclerosing cholangitis. Surg Gynecol Obstet 1993; 177(4):335–44.
11. Ghali P, Marotta PJ, Yoshida EM, et al. Liver transplantation for incidental cholangiocarcinoma: analysis of the Canadian experience. Liver Transpl 2005;11(11): 1412–6.
12. Meyer CG, Penn I, James L. Liver transplantation for cholangiocarcinoma: results in 207 patients. Transplantation 2000;69(8):1633–7.
13. Robles R, Figueras J, Turrion VS, et al. Spanish experience in liver transplantation for hilar and peripheral cholangiocarcinoma. Ann Surg 2004;239(2):265–71.
14. Becker NS, Rodriguez JA, Barshes NR, et al. Outcomes analysis for 280 patients with cholangiocarcinoma treated with liver transplantation over an 18-year period. J Gastrointest Surg 2008;12(1):117–22.
15. Pitt HA, Nakeeb A, Abrams RA, et al. Perihilar cholangiocarcinoma: postoperative radiotherapy does not improve survival. Ann Surg 1995;221(6):788–97 [discussion 797–8].
16. McMasters KM, Tuttle TM, Leach SD, et al. Neoadjuvant chemoradiation for extrahepatic cholangiocarcinoma. Am J Surg 1997;174(6):605–8 [discussion 608–9].
17. Alden ME, Mohiuddin M. The impact of radiation dose in combined external beam and intraluminal Ir-192 brachytherapy for bile duct cancer. Int J Radiat Oncol Biol Phys 1994;28(4):945–51.

18. Foo ML, Gunderson LL, Bender CE, et al. External radiation therapy and trans-catheter iridium in the treatment of extrahepatic bile duct carcinoma. Int J Radiat Oncol Biol Phys 1997;39(4):929–35.
19. Sudan D, DeRoover A, Chinnakotla S, et al. Radiochemotherapy and transplantation allow long-term survival for nonresectable hilar cholangiocarcinoma. Am J Transplant 2002;2(8):774–9.
20. Gleeson FC, Rajan E, Levy MJ, et al. EUS-guided FNA of regional lymph nodes in patients with unresectable hilar cholangiocarcinoma. Gastrointest Endosc 2008; 67(3):438–43.
21. De Vreede I, Steers JL, Burch PA, et al. Prolonged disease-free survival after orthotopic liver transplantation plus adjuvant chemoirradiation for cholangiocarcinoma. Liver Transpl 2000;6(3):309–16.
22. Rea DJ, Heimbach JK, Rosen CB, et al. Liver transplantation with neoadjuvant chemoradiation is more effective than resection for hilar cholangiocarcinoma. Ann Surg 2005;242(3):451–8 [discussion 458–61].
23. Heimbach JK, Gores GJ, Haddock MG, et al. Predictors of disease recurrence following neoadjuvant chemoradiotherapy and liver transplantation for unresectable perihilar cholangiocarcinoma. Transplantation 2006;82(12):1703–7.
24. Mantel HT, Rosen CB, Heimbach JK, et al. Vascular complications after orthotopic liver transplantation after neoadjuvant therapy for hilar cholangiocarcinoma. Liver Transpl 2007;13(10):1372–81.
25. Gores GJ, Gish RG, Sudan D, et al. Model for end-stage liver disease (MELD) exception for cholangiocarcinoma or biliary dysplasia. Liver Transpl 2006; 12(Suppl 12):S95–7.
26. Neuhaus P, Jonas S, Bechstein WO, et al. Extended resections for hilar cholangiocarcinoma. Ann Surg 1999;230(6):808–18 [discussion 819].
27. Jonas S, Benckert C, Thelen A, et al. Radical surgery for hilar cholangiocarcinoma. Eur J Surg Oncol 2008;34(3):263–71.

Radical Resection of Biliary Tract Cancers and the Role of Extended Lymphadenectomy

Yasuji Seyama, MD, PhD[a], Norihiro Kokudo, MD, PhD[a],
Masatoshi Makuuchi, MD, PhD[b],*

KEYWORDS

- Bile duct cancer • Lymphadenectomy
- Extended hemihepatectomy • Pancreatoduodenectomy
- Biliary drainage • Portal vein embolization

Extrahepatic bile duct (EBD) cancer is difficult to diagnose at an early stage and, consequently, EBD cancer is often found at an advanced stage after invasion or metastasis has occurred.[1–4] However, the long-term survival rates of patients who undergo surgery with curative intent is superior to the survival rates of patients who did not undergo resection; additionally, only resection offers a chance for a cure.[1,3–7] EBD resection alone is usually insufficient for a curative resection because EBD cancer spreads along the bile duct and invades adjacent structures. The surgical procedure is typically selected according to the tumor location.[1,8] A pancreatoduodenectomy (PD) and an extended hemihepatectomy have been proposed as standard procedures for the resection of distal and hilar bile duct cancer, respectively. Furthermore, extended radical procedures, including a right lobectomy, a left trisectoriectomy, hepatopancreatoduodenectomy, and combined resection of the portal vein or hepatic artery, have been reported to enable a negative surgical margin to be obtained. However, about two-thirds of patients with EBD cancer develop obstructive jaundice, which increases the operative risks. Thus, the risks and benefits of these extended radical operations should be carefully estimated. On the other hand, lymph node metastasis is commonly observed in patients with EBD cancer and has been described as a strong prognostic factor. Patterns of tumor that spread via the lymphatic route are also dependent on the tumor location.[9–11] The significance and

[a] Division of Hepato-Biliary-Pancreatic Surgery, Department of Surgery, Graduate School of Medicine, University of Tokyo, 7-3-1 Hongo, Bunkyo-ku, Tokyo 113-8655, Japan
[b] Department of Surgery, Japanese Red Cross Medical Center, 4-1-22 Hiro-o, Shibuya-ku, Tokyo 150-8935, Japan
* Corresponding author.
E-mail address: makuuchi_masatoshi@med.jrc.or.jp (M. Makuuchi).

Surg Oncol Clin N Am 18 (2009) 339–359
doi:10.1016/j.soc.2008.12.011
1055-3207/08/$ – see front matter © 2009 Elsevier Inc. All rights reserved.

surgonc.theclinics.com

adequate area of a lymphadenectomy for EBD cancer have been controversial. This article reviews the literature regarding EBD cancer and focuses on standard and extended surgical procedures, extended lymphadenectomy, short- and long-term outcome, and prognostic factors.

EXTRAHEPATIC BILE DUCT CANCER AND GROUPING OF REGIONAL LYMPH NODES

The term "cholangiocarcinoma" has recently been used to describe malignancies arising from both the intrahepatic and the extrahepatic bile duct.[3,4,8,12] Intrahepatic cholangiocarcinoma is usually treated as a primary liver cancer because the required surgical procedures are similar to hepatocellular carcinoma, ie, hepatic resection. This discussion focuses on the radical surgical treatment of EBD cancer, which is classified according to its location: hilar, middle, and distal bile duct (**Fig. 1**). Almost two-thirds of all cases of EBD cancer are located in the perihilar region and the reminders originate from the distal bile duct; however, the resection rate is higher for distal bile duct cancer than for hilar bile duct cancer.[1,8] Hilar bile duct cancer is further divided into four groups according to the Bismuth-Corlette classification, which is closely related to the surgical procedure that is ultimately selected (**Fig. 2**).[13,14]

EBD cancer easily metastasizes to the lymph nodes; the average rate of lymph node metastasis has been reported to be 41% (**Table 1**).[1,2,5–7,10,15–27] The presence of nodal metastasis has been described as a strong prognostic factor; therefore, an exact identification of the nodal status is important for biliary surgery. The regional lymph nodes of EBD include the nodes in the hepatoduodenal ligament (#12), around the pancreatic head (#13 and #17), along the common hepatic artery (#8), and along the superior mesenteric artery (#14); the lymph nodes groupings are classified according to the tumor's location (**Fig. 3A, B**).[28] Group 3 lymph nodes, including paraaortic nodes, are generally considered as distant metastases (**Fig. 3**).

In this article, the name of the hepatic area and the resections are based on Couinaud's segmentation.[29] For example, a right hemihepatectomy includes Couinaud's segments 5–8, while a right lobectomy means the resection of Couinaud's segments 4–8.

ASSESSMENT OF RESECTABILITY

The first steps in the diagnosis of EBD cancer are a blood biochemical examination and an abdominal ultrasonography; the next step is computed tomography (CT) and magnetic resonance (MR) imaging.[30,31] Direct cholangiography via an endoscopic or percutaneous route is an invasive work-up, but it provides useful information about the horizontal extension of EBD cancer. Resectability is assessed based on CT, MR imaging, and cholangiography findings. Contraindications for curative intent surgery are: the presence of distant metastasis including the paraaortic lymph nodes; invasion to the whole hepatoduodenal ligament; and bilateral spread beyond the second bifurcation of the intrahepatic bile duct. Vascular invasion requiring combined resection and reconstruction is not a contraindication but should be carefully considered when selecting patients.[32–35] Surgical procedures are selected according to the tumor location and the horizontal spread identified by direct cholangiography.[5,36–39]

MODE OF SPREAD OF BILE DUCT CANCER

The longitudinal extension of bile duct cancer is usually beyond the macroscopic or cholangioscopic border, and the mode of extension is characterized by superficial spreading or submucosal invasion.[40–42] Superficial spreading is predominantly seen in papillary or nodular-type.[41]Yamaguchi and colleagues[40] reported that the mean

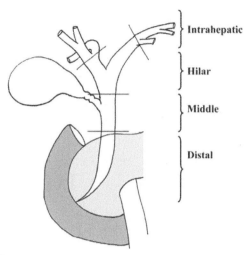

Intrahepatic

Hilar

Middle

Distal

Fig. 1. Schema of biliary tract.

distance between the macroscopic and microscopic edge was 6.1 mm in the hepatic and 6.2 mm in the duodenal direction. Sakamoto and colleagues[41] documented that the mucosal extension was within 5 mm in 8 of 17 patients but greater than 20 mm in 8 of 17 patients. On the other hand, submucosal invasion extends via the lymphatic, perineural, or venous vessels, and it is predominant in the flat or nodular infiltrating types of cancer.[40–42] The length of microscopic submucosal extension beyond the macroscopic edge was limited to 10 mm.[40,42] A tumor-free margin less than 5 mm was closely associated with early of local recurrence.[41,43] Thus, a macroscopic surgical margin of over 10 mm is desirable for infiltrating-type cancer, while a margin of over 20 mm is necessary for papillary and nodular-types of cancer. The intraoperative pathologic examination of frozen sections is advocated to obtain a negative surgical margin. Additional resection should be performed if the site is the only positive margin.

Hilar bile duct cancer frequently invades vertically to the right hepatic artery, portal vein, hepatic parenchyma, and gallbladder. Distal bile duct cancer tends to infiltrate the pancreatic parenchyma, the duodenum, and the portal vein. A hepatectomy for hilar bile duct cancer and a PD for distal bile duct cancer are needed to obtain a curative resection.[5,8,36,37,39,44–46]

PREOPERATIVE TREATMENT: BILIARY DRAINAGE

Preoperative biliary drainage has been performed to improve liver function and to reduce operative risk because of the high rate of obstructive jaundice in patients with EBD cancer.[47–54] However, the benefit of preoperative biliary drainage has not been proven using comparative studies, and the complications arising from the procedures, including the occurrence of cholangitis, tract seeding, and the risk of pancreatitis, have been emphasized.[55–58] Biliary drainage before PD without hepatectomy is not always performed, in view of the benefits and drawbacks. In contrast, biliary drainage before hepatectomy has been advocated because of the risk of postoperative liver failure.[5,39,54,55,58–60] Biliary drainage before major hepatectomy has been routinely performed in patients with hilar bile duct cancer according to the reports from high volume centers published in the twenty first century **(Table 2)**.[5,6,21–27,61–63]

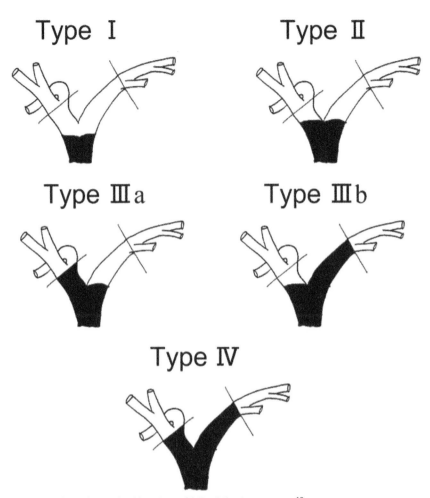

Fig. 2. Bismuth-Corlette classification of hilar bile duct cancer.[13]

Seyama and colleagues[39] described the principles of preoperative biliary drainage: the advantage of returning the externally drained bile juice by oral intake,[64] the sufficient functional recovery of jaundiced liver,[5,36,37] the need for biliary drainage before hepatectomy,[47,48,54,59] the periodic exchange of endoscopic retrograde biliary drainage stent tubes,[65,66] and the need for bile cultures and isolation using tests for antibiotics sensitivity.[67] If the right and left hepatic duct are separated by the invasion of hilar bile duct cancer, percutaneous transhepatic biliary drainage (PTBD) for only the future remnant liver is the first choice.[5,23,68–70] Hemihepatic biliary drainage is sufficient to enable liver dysfunction caused by obstructive jaundice to recover.[68,69,71] The endoscopic route is not advocated for hilar bile duct cancer of Bismuth type 2–4 because of the high incidence of cholangitis in the undrained area.[65,72–74] Even in patients who have Bismuth type 1, the possibility of cholangitits of undrained hepatic areas, such as isolated bifurcations of the posterior bile duct, should be considered. Direct cholangiography should be limited to the time of the initial puncture and the day before the operation; the resulting information is sufficient to perform an extended hemihepatectomy for hilar bile duct cancer.[5,39] Biliary

Table 1
Literature review of bile duct cancer and lymph node metastasis

Author	Year	Site of Tumor	pN+/Total	Rate of pN+ (%)	Median Survival (Months)			5-year Survival Rate (%)				Mortality Rate %	Mortality in OS
					pN0	pN1	pN2	pN0	pN1	pN2	OS		
Todoroki[15]	2001	Distal	35/52	67%	—	—	—	61	41	9	39	5	included
Nagakawa[1]	2002	Distal	627/1543	40%	—	—	—	35	17	10	26	NA	NA
Yoshida[16]	2002	Distal	15/27	58%	—	—	—	61	20	—	—	4	excluded
Sakamoto[17]	2005	Distal	27/51	53%	38	27	—	42	16	—	24	7	included
Cheng Q[18]	2007	Distal	25/112	22%	46	13	—	30	4	—	25	3	excluded
Murakami[19]	2007	Distal	16/36	44%	—	—	—	73	17	—	50	0	no mortality
Hong[20]	2005	EHBD	68/209	33%	44	20[a]	—	—	—	—	—	NA	NA
Jang[7]	2005	EHBD	36/151	24%	29	13	14[b]	—	—	—	33	3	included
Schwarz[2]	2007	EHBD	150/393	38%	37	16	—	40	14	—	22	7	included
Todoroki[21]	2000	Hilar	46/98	46%	41	26	11	39	29	6	28	4	included
Jarnagin[22]	2001	Hilar	19/80	24%	42	39	—	—	—	—	39	10	included
Kitagawa[10]	2001	Hilar	58/110	53%	—	—	—	31	15	—	—	10	—
Nagakawa[1]	2002	Hilar	514/1183	45%	—	—	—	29	15	11	26	NA	NA
Kawasaki[23]	2003	Hilar	35/78	45%	54	24	—	42	16	—	40	1	included
Seyama[5]	2003	Hilar	28/58	52%	80	24	15	67	23	10	40	0	no mortality
Rea[24]	2004	Hilar	8/46	17%	34	15	—	27	12	—	—	9	included
Hemming[6]	2005	Hilar	NA	NA	—	—	—	45	21	—	35	9	included
Dinant[25]	2006	Hilar	23/99	23%	42	18	—	—	—	—	27	15	included
Baton[26]	2007	Hilar	30/59	51%	—	—	—	31	13	—	20	5	included
Hasegawa[27]	2007	Hilar	17/49	35%	60	25	—	46	27	—	40	2	included

Abbreviations: distal, distal bile duct cancer; EHBD, extrahepatic bile duct cancer; hilar, hilar bile duct cancer; pN, microscopic lymph node metastasis; pN2, group 2 lymph node metastasis.
[a] pN1 represent patients with 1–4 lymph node metastases.
[b] pN2 means patients with 5 or more lymph node metastases.

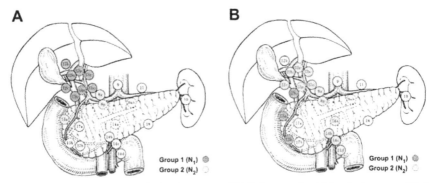

Fig. 3. Regional lymph node of bile duct cancer[28] (*A*) for proximal bile duct cancer; (*B*) for distal bile duct cancer. (*Red circle*) Group 1 (N_1). (*Yellow circle*), Group 2 (N_2). (*White circle*), Group 3 (N_3). *From* Japanese Society of Biliary Surgery. Classification of biliary tract carcinoma. 2nd English edition. Tokyo: Kanehara; 2004; with permission.

drainage before hepatectomy is scheduled before portal vein embolization as a part of safe treatment strategy for hilar bile duct cancer.[5]

PREOPERATIVE TREATMENT: PORTAL VEIN EMBOLIZATION

Preoperative portal vein embolization (PVE) is a useful option to prevent liver failure after hepatic resection. Makuuchi and colleagues[75,76] reported the first series of PVE for hilar cholangiocarcinoma enabling extended hemihepatectomies to be safely performed. The effect of PVE has been confirmed in a meta-analysis; the rate of liver failure after major hepatic resection has decreased from 2.5% to 0.8% as a result of PVE.[77] The rate of liver failure and mortality after a major hepatectomy for hilar cholangiocarcinoma has also been reduced by PVE (see **Table 2**).[39] Previously proposed indication criteria for PVE were based on the volume of the future remnant liver, as estimated using computed tomography.[5,78–80] Because assessments of liver function before hepatectomy are difficult in patients who have jaundice,[81] a safe strategy for patients with hilar bile duct cancer was proposed (**Fig. 4**).[5] In patients who have normal liver function, PVE is indicated when the future remnant liver is less than 40%. In patients with obstructive jaundice, PVE is scheduled following biliary drainage if the future remnant liver is estimated to be less than 50%. This strategy seems to provide safe indications, resulting in no mortality.[5] The wider indications for PVE than for an right hemihepatectomy for liver tumors in terms of ICG are because of the resection of the lower part of segment 4 and the caudate lobe in patients who have liver damage caused by obstructive jaundice.

SURGICAL TREATMENTS FOR HILAR BILE DUCT CANCER

Considering the horizontal and vertical extension of the bile duct cancer, EBD resection with a hepatectomy, including a caudate lobectomy and regional lymphadenectomy, is the best treatment for hilar bile duct cancer. Hepatectomy has increased the resectability and curability rates for hilar bile duct cancer, as described in literature reviews.[39,82] The caudate lobe is easily invaded by the hilar bile duct cancer because the orifice of the caudate bile duct usually opens in the hilar bile duct.[83–87] A caudate lobectomy is therefore necessary for a curative resection of hilar bile duct cancer; its safety and impact on long-term survival has been reported.[87–89] Liu and colleagues[62] pointed out that improved long-term outcomes partially depended on the routine use

Table 2
Literature review of preoperative treatment for hilar bile duct cancer

Author	Year	Major Hx	BD	PVE	Liver Failure	Mortality
Todoroki[21]	2000	32	Done	No	8%	5%
Cherqui[63]	2000	20	No	No	5%	5%
Jarnagin[22]	2001	62	Not routine	No	3%	11%
Seyama[5]	2003	58	Done	Done	0%	0%
Kawasaki[23]	2003	69	Done	Done	0%	1%
Rea[24]	2004	46	Done	No	11%	9%
Kondo[61]	2004	26	Done	Done	0%	0%
Hemming[6]	2005	52	Done	Done	4%	9%
Dinant[25]	2006	38	Done	No	10%	15%
Liu[62]	2006	38	Done	No→done	8%	20%
Baton[26]	2007	58	Done	No→done	3%	5%
Hasegawa[27]	2007	44	Done	No	14%	2%

Abbreviations: BD, biliary drainage; Hx, hepatectomy; PVE, portal vein embolization.

of a total caudate lobectomy. Tsao and colleagues[90] compared the surgical outcomes for hilar bile duct caner between 25 cases at the Lahey Clinic in the United States and 122 cases at Nagoya University Hospital in Japan; they showed that the rates of liver resection, caudate lobectomy, curative resection, and 5-year survival rate were 89%, 89%, 79%, and 16% in the Nagoya cohort and 16%, 8%, 28%, and 8% in the Lahey cohort, respectively. Liver resection with a caudate lobectomy contributed to the higher rates of curative resection and long-term survival.

EXTENDED HEMIHEPATECTOMY

An extended hemihepatectomy is a standard hepatectomy procedure because of its curability and simplicity.[5,22,23,36,37,39,61,82,91,92] The choice of a right or left hemihepatectomy is made according to the tumor location, based on ultrasonography and CT findings, because hemihepatic biliary drainage for only the future remnant liver is desirable for patients who have separated hepatic ducts, such as patients with Bismuth type 2–4 tumors.[5,13,14,39] An extended right hepatectomy is performed if the tumor is located on the right side or centrally, and the resection area includes the right liver, inferior part of Couinaud's segment 4, and the whole caudate lobe. The resection line of the liver and the transected surface is shown in **Fig. 5**. The right side of the umbilical fossa is dissected free, and the hilar plate is cut at the right edge of the umbilical portion (**Fig. 5**).[23] An extended left hepatectomy is elected if the tumor location is left-side dominant and if the resection area includes the left liver, hilar part of the right paramedian sector, and the whole caudate lobe (**Fig. 6**). Yamanaka and colleagues[93] reported that 11 patients underwent a left hemihepatectomy with reconstruction of eight portal veins and nine right hepatic arteries; the short-term results were better, but the long-term survivals were worse in those patients than in 14 patients who underwent a right hemihepatectomy. Left hemihepatectomy with reconstruction of the right hepatic artery is an option for patients in whom an extended right hepatectomy would be regarded as a high-risk procedure.

RIGHT LOBECTOMY OR LEFT TRISECTORIECTOMY

A right lobectomy (resection of segments 4–8) or a left trisectoriectomy (resection of segments 2–5 and 8) is a more aggressive treatment for hilar bile duct cancer of

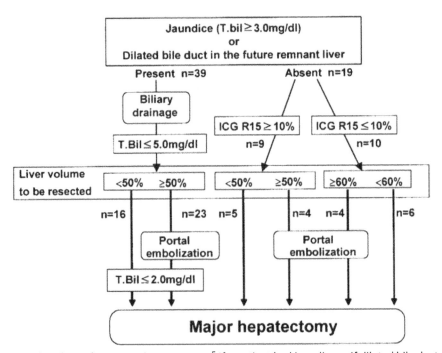

Fig. 4. Flowchart of preoperative treatment.[5] If a patient had jaundice or if dilated bile ducts were present in the future remnant liver, biliary drainage (BD) was performed. Surgical interventions were scheduled after the hepatic function had sufficiently recovered. Portal vein embolization (PVE) was performed to avoid postoperative liver failure, depending on the liver function and the liver volume to be resected. *From* Seyama Y, Kubota K, Sano K, et al. Long-term outcome of extended hemihepatectomy for hilar bile duct cancer with no mortality and high survival rate. Ann Surg 2003;238(1):73–83; with permission.

Bismuth type 4 than an extended hemihepatectomy, but these procedures enable a surgical margin to be obtained in the hepatic direction.[76,94–98] However, the risks of postoperative liver failure and death are also increased because the remnant liver is only two segments. A right lobectomy may provide a negative surgical margin even in patients with advanced hilar bile duct cancer because the transection point of the left hepatic duct is the left side of the umbilical part, including the adjacent liver parenchyma.[95,98] However, the remnant liver comprises only segments 2 and 3, and portal vein embolization of the right lobe is mandatory to prevent liver failure.[94,96] Nagino and colleagues[98] reported that eight patients who had hilar bile duct cancer underwent a right lobectomy with a negative hepatic margin rate of 87.5% (7/8), but the liver failure rate was 25% (2/8). Moreover, patients who had lymph node metastasis died within three years as a result of tumor recurrence. A right lobectomy may enable long-term survival for selected patients who have locally advanced tumors without nodal metastasis, but the high risk of liver failure must be considered when determining the surgical indications. On the other hand, Makuuchi and colleagues[76] reported the first-ever successful left trisectoriectomy for hilar bile duct cancer after portal vein embolization. Shimada and colleagues[97] reported 12 cases of left trisectoriectomy; the incidence of curative resection was 75% with no mortality after biliary drainage and portal vein embolization. If the posterior branch originates from the

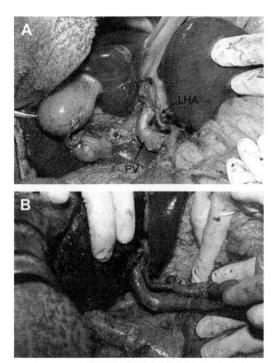

Fig. 5. Intraoperative view of extended right hepatectomy. (*A*) Visceral surface after skeltonization of the hepatoduodenal ligament. The right side of the umbilical part is dissected. The transection line is marked on the liver using electrocautery. (*B*) Raw surface of the liver after extended right hepatectomy. The three stumps of the bile duct in the umbilical fossa are visible. The left hepatic duct has been completely removed.

common hepatic duct or left hepatic duct, a tumor-free margin may be long when performing resection by left trisectoriectomy.[39]

INDICATION OF HEPATOPANCREATODUODENECTOMY

Hepatopancreatoduodenectomy (HPD) is a useful option for obtaining negative margins in patients who have widely spread bile duct cancer where the tumor extends from the hilar to the intrapancreatic bile duct.[5,23,38,99–101] HPD offers the possibility of long-term survival to patients who have widely spread bile duct cancer and without lymph node metastasis, if a negative surgical margin is obtained.[100–103] HPD is not advocated for the purpose of removing extensive lymph node metastasis because of the poor patient prognosis. HPD for bile duct cancer usually consists of an extended right hepatectomy with PD; a high mortality rate (14%–35%) has been reported.[99,101–104] In a series of 58 patients who had HPD performed over a period of 23 years, Ebata and colleagues[102] reported that the mortality rate remained constant at 14% (2/14) despite improvements in the rates of liver failure and pancreatic leakage, even in the twenty first century. Preoperative biliary drainage followed by PVE is necessary to prevent postoperative liver failure, but pancreatic leakage is another problem associated with HPD which can cause postoperative bleeding from the major arteries resulting in mortality. A two-stage pancreatojejunostomy with an omental patch has been reported to reduce the risk of pancreatic leakage and mortality as a result of PD; this technique is advocated, especially in high-risk patients.[105–108] In

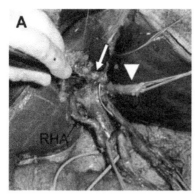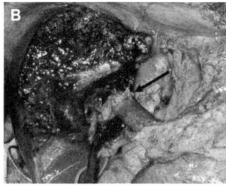

Fig. 6. Intraoperative view of extended hemihepatectomy for hilar bile duct cancer. (*A*) The bifurcation of the portal vein has been invaded by the tumor (*white arrow*); the umbilical portion of the portal vein is dissected free and used as a venous graft (*white arrowhead*). (*B*) A venous patch is used to reconstruct the bifurcation of the portal vein (*arrow*).

the two-stage method, the pancreatic juice is externally drained at the time of the PD and a pancreatojejunostomy is completed about three months later.[105,106] A two-stage pancreatojejunostomy with an omental patch may reduce the risk of bleeding from arteries; no mortalities have been reported in series where this technique was used together with biliary drainage and PVE.[5,100,105]

COMBINED VASCULAR RESECTION AND RECONSTRUCTION

Combined portal vein resection and reconstruction—together with an extended hemihepatectomy—have been reported as useful for the treatment of locally advanced hilar bile duct cancer with its high mortality rate (9%–40%).[32,33,35,70,109,110] Recent studies have shown that an extended hemihepatectomy with portal vein resection can be safely performed using preoperative PVE.[5,23,61] Previous large series have shown that the survival rate of patients with combined portal vein resection is worse than that of patients without portal vein resection.[32,33,35] However, there have been long-term survivors among the selected patients with portal vein resection with a negative margin and without lymph node metastasis.[35] Ebata and colleagues[32] reported that 52 patients underwent combined portal vein resection because of gross tumor invasion and that microscopic invasion was found in 36 of them (69%). Severe adhesion and tumor invasion is hard to distinguish intraoperatively, but the distance between the tumor and portal vein is too small to dissect without exposure. A combined portal vein resection should be indicated when the site is the only obstacle for a curative resection, regardless of the pathologic proof. Intraoperative views of patients undergoing an extended left hepatectomy with portal vein resection have shown that the umbilical part of the portal vein can be harvested and used to reconstruct the bifurcation of the portal vein (**Fig. 6**A, B).

Combined resection and reconstruction of the hepatic artery of the remnant liver is reported to be associated with a high morality and a low survival rate in patients with hilar cholangiocarcinoma.[32–35,93] Miyazaki and colleagues[35] reported that nine patients underwent combined hepatic artery resection and reconstruction with various type of hepatectomy procedures; the mortality rate was 33% (3/9), and the remaining six patients died within three years. Sakamoto and colleagues[34] reported that four patients with hilar bile duct cancer underwent combined resection and reconstruction of the right hepatic artery with no mortalities, but all the patients died within two years.

Additionally, the long-term survival rates of patients who underwent the simultaneous resection and reconstruction of both the portal vein and the hepatic artery together with a hepatectomy were significantly worse than those of patients undergoing resection and reconstruction of the portal vein alone.[34,35] According to these reports, there has been no evidence to indicate a benefit of the combined resection and reconstruction of the hepatic artery of the remnant liver on patient survival.

More extensive resections aimed to non-touch technique have also been reported. Mimura and colleagues[104] reported six cases of hepatoligamentectomy for bile duct cancer, in which the portal vein and hepatic artery were routinely resected en bloc with the surrounding tissues, together with a PD in four patients and a hemihepatectomy in two patients, but the mortality rate was 33% (2/6). Neuhaus and colleagues[70] reported that a hemihepatectomy with portal vein resection and reconstruction was performed in 23 patients with: a mortality rate of 17% (4/23); a curative resection rate of 61% (14/23); and microscopic portal vein invasion in 22% (5/23). They suggested that portal vein resection was an effective "no-touch technique;" however, the benefit was limited and the risk was high. Considering the high mortality rate, the use of combined vascular resection as a no-touch technique is not justified.

SURGICAL TREATMENT FOR MIDDLE BILE DUCT CANCER

Middle bile duct cancer is usually treated by a PD. If the tumor extension is predominantly to the hilar side, an extended hemihepatectomy is the choice of treatment. EBD resection alone is not advocated because of the high rate of positive margins, compared with combined resections of the pancreas or liver,[111] and EBD resection is an option only for patients with papillary tumors limited to the middle bile duct without lymph node metastasis or for patients for whom a radical resection would be a high-risk procedure.[7] An extended extrahepatic resection, in which the intrapancreatic bile duct is excavated as a 2–3 cm long funnel, has been reported to be beneficial to patients who have a high operative risk to avoid the need for a PD.[112]

SURGICAL TREATMENT FOR DISTAL BILE DUCT CANCER

PD is a standard surgical treatment for distal bile duct cancer.[45] Pylorus-preserving PD (PpPD) is widely performed; randomized clinical trials have shown little difference between PpPD and conventional PD with regard to both short-term and long-term results.[113–117] PD with portal vein resection has not been applied to patients with distal bile duct cancer but has been applied to patients with pancreatic head cancer; a survival benefit has only been indicated among selected patients with curative resections.[118] As the distance between the intrapancreatic bile duct and the portal vein is not negligible, distal bile duct cancer, which requires combined portal vein resection, is regarded as a locally advanced tumor.

ROLE OF EXTENDED LYMPHADENECTOMY FOR EBD CANCER

Lymph node metastasis is commonly observed among patients who have bile duct cancer and it has been reported as a strong prognostic factor for long-term outcome after curative intent surgery. The long-term outcome of the patients with nodal metastasis was worse than that of patients without nodal metastasis (see **Table 1**). Especially, the 5-year survival rate of patients with metastasis to the second group of lymph nodes (pN2) was about 10% (see **Table 1**). The purposes of extended lymphadenectomy for bile duct cancer are to remove the local tumor spread via the lymphatic route and to enable accurate staging.

The pattern of lymphatic spread differs according to the location of the primary tumor; consequently, the appropriate area of an extended regional lymphadenectomy also differs similarly.[9–11] Hilar bile duct cancer spreads from the lymph nodes in the hepatoduodenal ligament (#12), which is the first and most frequent metastatic station (group 1, N1), along the common hepatic artery (#8) or to the superior retropancreatic nodes (#13a) (group 2, N2, **Fig. 2B**).[11] Skeltonization of the hepatoduodenal ligament and clearance of the soft tissues of the superior retropancreatic area and along the common hepatic artery are mandatory for curative intent surgery for hilar bile duct cancer (**Figs. 6 and 7**).[5] On the other hand, middle and distal bile duct cancer extends from the nodes behind the pancreatic head (#13) to the nodes around the superior mesenteric artery (#14) or from the nodes in the hepatoduodenal ligament (#12b, a, p) to the nodes along the common hepatic artery (#8); therefore, PD with skeltonization of the hepatoduodenal ligament and dissection of the right side of the superior mesenteric artery, which includes both group 1 and 2 lymph nodes (see **Fig. 3**), has been advocated.[9,16] As mentioned above, the appropriate area for an extended lymphadenectomy for bile duct cancer is considered to include the region up to the group 2 lymph nodes.

An extended retroperitoneal lymphadenectomy, including dissection of the paraaortic lymph nodes, for the treatment of EBD cancer has been tried by some aggressive surgeons.[9,10] Yeo and colleagues[46,119,120] reported that an extended lymphadenectomy did not influence either the short-term or long-term results after PD among 296 cases with periampullary malignancies, including 51 cases with distal bile duct cancer, regardless of whether lymph node metastasis was present or absent in a randomized controlled study. In general, paraaortic lymph node metastasis from hilar bile duct cancer has been considered as a distant metastasis, and the prognosis of such patients has been regarded as poor. Kitagawa and colleagues[10] reported that paraaortic lymph nodes were pathologically detected in 19 of 110 patients (17.3%) with hilar bile duct cancer; two of seven patients who had only microscopic metastasis survived for more than 5 years, but the remaining 12 patients who had macroscopic metastasis died within 2 years. The group also insisted that extended lymph node dissection was not effective for patients who had widespread nodal involvement but might benefit patients who had regional node metastasis. As mentioned above, no

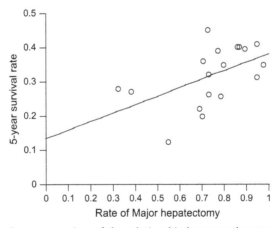

Fig. 7. Data from a literature review of the relationship between the rate of major hepatectomy and the 5-year survival rate. Linear approximation showed a significant correlation ($P = .0274$, R = 0.52).

evidence suggested that an extended retroperitoneal lymphadenectomy may influence the long-term survival of patients who had EBD cancer.

IMPACT OF THE NUMBER OF RETRIEVED AND METASTATIC LYMPH NODES

Recently, the total number of dissected lymph nodes has also become a matter of interest. For gastric, colorectal, and pancreatic cancer, the total number of lymph nodes analyzed has been reported to be an important predictor of long-term survival, although the impact of stage migration effect and regional disease control has not been determined.[121–126] For colon and pancreatic cancer, a minimum of 12 lymph nodes are required for the accurate diagnosis of a negative lymph node status.[121,125] Long-term survival improved as more lymph nodes were analyzed in patients with gastric or colon cancer, and the total number of retrieved lymph nodes itself was a prognostic variable.[123,124]

For EBD cancer, Hong and colleagues[20] reported that there was no survival difference according to the total number of retrieved lymph nodes when a mean of 11 lymph nodes were analyzed. In contrast, Schwarz and colleagues[2] reported that the mean number of dissected lymph nodes was only four when based on United States population data and the total lymph node count influenced long-term survival irrespective of the pathologic nodal status. They also proposed that 10 or more lymph nodes should be examined for curative intent resections for EBD cancer. On the other hand, the mean number of total dissected lymph nodes for EBD cancer has been reported to be 24 to 32 according to the reports from Japan; consequently the long-term outcome is superior to that in other countries.[10,11,19] Considering the results of these reports, an extended lymphadenectomy of the regional nodes for EBD cancer is necessary for curative intent surgery, and at least 10 or more lymph nodes should be examined to obtain an accurate staging.

The number of positive lymph nodes has been reported to be an important surrogate marker of the tumor staging; the UICC classification of gastric and colon cancer includes the number of positive nodes when grouping the regional lymph node status.[127] The impact of the number of positive nodes on long-term outcome has also been studied for EDB cancer. Yoshida and colleagues[11] examined the relationship between the number of cancer-positive lymph nodes and the long-term outcome after PD for distal BD cancer and showed that patients with three or more positive nodes had a significantly worse outcome. Murakami and colleagues[19] also reported that there were no long-term survivors among the patients with three or more lymph node metastases. Hong and colleagues[20] reported that the prognosis of patients with five or more metastatic lymph nodes was significantly worse than that of patients with fewer than four positive nodes. Thus, the cut-off for survival seems to be three to five positive nodes. In other words, there is a chance of long-term survival among patients with two or fewer involved lymph nodes, although the presence of lymph node metastasis is negative prognostic factor.

RESULTS OF SURGICAL TREATMENT AND PROGNOSTIC FACTORS

The long-term outcome of patients with EBD cancer has been improved as a result of the radical surgical treatments mentioned above; recent reports have shown that the 5-year survival rates after curative intent surgery ranged from 24% to 50% for patients with distal bile duct cancer and from 26% to 40% for patients with hilar bile duct cancer (see **Table 1**). A reduction in operative mortality is important for improving surgical outcome. The mortality rate of hilar bile duct cancer has been reported to be higher than that of distal bile duct cancer (see **Table 1**). Perioperative deaths are sometimes excluded to elucidate the prognostic factors influencing long-term survival;[16,18] however, the overall survival rate, including perioperative mortality, is essential for determining the impact of surgical treatment for malignancies. For hilar bile duct cancer, the positive correlations between the hepatectomy and resectability rates and between the major hepatectomy and curative resection rates have been pointed out.[39,82] As a result, the 5-year survival rate after the resection of hilar bile duct cancer has improved as more major hepatectomies have been performed (see **Fig. 7**). Jang and colleagues[7] followed the clinical course after the resection of 151 cases of EBD cancer and showed that 49 patients had survived for more than 5 years, but late recurrences after 5 years occurred in 8 patients and long-term follow up was necessary to declare "a cure."

Residual tumor status, lymph node metastasis, tumor differentiation, tumor size, tumor stage, blood transfusion, and operative time have been reported as significant prognostic factors.[5,7–9,15,17,20,22,24,26,62,70,91,92,119,128–130] Lymph node metastasis has been shown to be the strongest prognostic factor, as revealed by multivariate analyses.[5,7,9,16,18,27,32,128,129] The surgical margin is also a strong prognostic factor, but multivariate analyses sometimes do not select this parameter. A positive margin involves two aspects, ie, the bile duct margin and the dissected margin. Sakamoto and colleagues[17] reported that a radical margin was more beneficial to the long-term outcome than the hepatic margin of the bile duct patients who have middle and distal bile duct cancer. Wakai and colleagues reported that invasive ductal carcinoma at the ductal resection margins was a strong negative prognostic factor, but residual carcinoma in situ was not. The significance of the hepatic or duodenal ductal margin status is still controversial, but additional resection should be performed if other factors, such as lymph node metastasis or the dissected margin, are hopeful for the patient's long-term survival. Blood loss of more than 1.5 L, the use of blood transfusion, and an operative time of more than 5 hours have been reported as adverse factors for long-term survival.[17,18,62] Blood loss procedures are also required for extended radical surgery.

Adjuvant chemotherapy was identified as a prognostic factor in a multivariate analysis by Yoshida et al[16]; however, the effect of adjuvant chemotherapy has not been determined for EBD cancer. The establishment of adjuvant therapy for long-term survival in high-risk patients, such as patients with nodal metastasis, positive margins, or combined vascular resections, is a future problem.

SUMMARY

Extended hemihepatectomy and/or PD plus EBD resection and an extended lymphadenectomy of up to the group 2 lymph nodes can enable long-term survival in patients with EBD cancer with acceptable surgical risks. Surgeons should dissect and examine at least 10 or more nodes in curative intent surgeries for local disease control and accurate staging. Radical surgical procedures for EBD cancer, including a right lobectomy, left trisectoriectomy, hepatopancreatoduodenectomy, and combined vascular resection and reconstruction, are useful options for obtaining a negative margin, but the benefits of such procedures to long-term survival rates is limited to selected patients without nodal metastasis and with negative surgical margins.

REFERENCES

1. Nagakawa T, Kayahara M, Ikeda S, et al. Biliary tract cancer treatment: results from the Biliary Tract Cancer Statistics Registry in Japan. J Hepatobiliary Pancreat Surg 2002;9(5):569–75.

2. Schwarz RE, Smith DD. Lymph node dissection impact on staging and survival of extrahepatic cholangiocarcinomas, based on U.S. population data. J Gastrointest Surg 2007;11(2):158–65.
3. de Groen PC, Gores GJ, LaRusso NF, et al. Biliary tract cancers. N Engl J Med 1999;341(18):1368–78.
4. Lazaridis KN, Gores GJ. Cholangiocarcinoma. Gastroenterology 2005;128(6): 1655–67.
5. Seyama Y, Kubota K, Sano K, et al. Long-term outcome of extended hemihepatectomy for hilar bile duct cancer with no mortality and high survival rate. Ann Surg 2003;238(1):73–83.
6. Hemming AW, Reed AI, Fujita S, et al. Surgical management of hilar cholangiocarcinoma. Ann Surg 2005;241(5):693–9 [discussion: 699–702].
7. Jang JY, Kim SW, Park DJ, et al. Actual long-term outcome of extrahepatic bile duct cancer after surgical resection. Ann Surg 2005;241(1):77–84.
8. Nakeeb A, Pitt HA, Sohn TA, et al. Cholangiocarcinoma. A spectrum of intrahepatic, perihilar, and distal tumors. Ann Surg 1996;224(4):463–73 [discussion: 473–5].
9. Kayahara M, Nagakawa T, Ohta T, et al. Role of nodal involvement and the periductal soft-tissue margin in middle and distal bile duct cancer. Ann Surg 1999; 229(1):76–83.
10. Kitagawa Y, Nagino M, Kamiya J, et al. Lymph node metastasis from hilar cholangiocarcinoma: audit of 110 patients who underwent regional and paraaortic node dissection. Ann Surg 2001;233(3):385–92.
11. Yoshida T, Matsumoto T, Sasaki A, et al. Lymphatic spread differs according to tumor location in extrahepatic bile duct cancer. Hepatogastroenterology 2003; 50(49):17–20.
12. Kokudo N, Makuuchi M. Extent of resection and outcome after curative resection for intrahepatic cholangiocarcinoma. Surg Oncol Clin N Am 2002;11(4):969–83.
13. Bismuth H, Corlette MB. Intrahepatic cholangioenteric anastomosis in carcinoma of the hilus of the liver. Surg Gynecol Obstet 1975;140(2):170–8.
14. Bismuth H, Nakache R, Diamond T. Management strategies in resection for hilar cholangiocarcinoma. Ann Surg 1992;215(1):31–8.
15. Todoroki T, Kawamoto T, Koike N, et al. Treatment strategy for patients with middle and lower third bile duct cancer. Br J Surg 2001;88(3):364–70.
16. Yoshida T, Matsumoto T, Sasaki A, et al. Prognostic factors after pancreatoduodenectomy with extended lymphadenectomy for distal bile duct cancer. Arch Surg 2002;137(1):69–73.
17. Sakamoto Y, Kosuge T, Shimada K, et al. Prognostic factors of surgical resection in middle and distal bile duct cancer: an analysis of 55 patients concerning the significance of ductal and radial margins. Surgery 2005;137(4):396–402.
18. Cheng Q, Luo X, Zhang B, et al. Distal bile duct carcinoma: prognostic factors after curative surgery. A series of 112 cases. Ann Surg Oncol 2007;14(3): 1212–9.
19. Murakami Y, Uemura K, Hayashidani Y, et al. Pancreatoduodenectomy for distal cholangiocarcinoma: prognostic impact of lymph node metastasis. World J Surg 2007;31(2):337–42 [discussion: 343–4].
20. Hong SM, Cho H, Lee OJ, et al. The number of metastatic lymph nodes in extrahepatic bile duct carcinoma as a prognostic factor. Am J Surg Pathol 2005; 29(9):1177–83.
21. Todoroki T, Kawamoto T, Koike N, et al. Radical resection of hilar bile duct carcinoma and predictors of survival. Br J Surg 2000;87(3):306–13.

22. Jarnagin WR, Fong Y, DeMatteo RP, et al. Staging, resectability, and outcome in 225 patients with hilar cholangiocarcinoma. Ann Surg 2001;234(4):507–17 [discussion: 517–9].
23. Kawasaki S, Imamura H, Kobayashi A, et al. Results of surgical resection for patients with hilar bile duct cancer: application of extended hepatectomy after biliary drainage and hemihepatic portal vein embolization. Ann Surg 2003; 238(1):84–92.
24. Rea DJ, Munoz-Juarez M, Farnell MB, et al. Major hepatic resection for hilar cholangiocarcinoma: analysis of 46 patients. Arch Surg 2004;139(5):514–23 [discussion: 523–5].
25. Dinant S, Gerhards MF, Rauws EA, et al. Improved outcome of resection of hilar cholangiocarcinoma (Klatskin tumor). Ann Surg Oncol 2006;13(6):872–80.
26. Baton O, Azoulay D, Adam DV, et al. Major hepatectomy for hilar cholangiocarcinoma type 3 and 4: prognostic factors and longterm outcomes. J Am Coll Surg 2007;204(2):250–60.
27. Hasegawa S, Ikai I, Fujii H, et al. Surgical resection of hilar cholangiocarcinoma: analysis of survival and postoperative complications. World J Surg 2007;31(6): 1256–63.
28. Japanese Society of Biliary Surgery. Classification of biliary tract carcinoma. 2nd English edition. Tokyo: Kanehara; 2004.
29. Couinaud C. Surgical anatomy of the liver revisted. Couinaud: Paris; 1989.
30. Miyakawa S, Ishihara S, Takada T, et al. Flowcharts for the management of biliary tract and ampullary carcinomas. J Hepatobiliary Pancreat Surg 2008;15(1): 7–14.
31. Zhong L, Xiao SD, Stoker J, et al. Magnetic resonance cholangiopancreatography. Chin J Dig Dis 2004;5(4):139–48.
32. Ebata T, Nagino M, Kamiya J, et al. Hepatectomy with portal vein resection for hilar cholangiocarcinoma: audit of 52 consecutive cases. Ann Surg 2003; 238(5):720–7.
33. Shimada H, Endo I, Sugita M, et al. Hepatic resection combined with portal vein or hepatic artery reconstruction for advanced carcinoma of the hilar bile duct and gallbladder. World J Surg 2003;27(10):1137–42.
34. Sakamoto Y, Sano T, Shimada K, et al. Clinical significance of reconstruction of the right hepatic artery for biliary malignancy. Langenbecks Arch Surg 2006; 391(3):203–8.
35. Miyazaki M, Kato A, Ito H, et al. Combined vascular resection in operative resection for hilar cholangiocarcinoma: does it work or not? Surgery 2007;141(5): 581–8.
36. Kawasaki S, Makuuchi M, Miyagawa S, et al. Radical operation after portal embolization for tumor of hilar bile duct. J Am Coll Surg 1994;178(5):480–6.
37. Miyagawa S, Makuuchi M, Kawasaki S. Outcome of extended right hepatectomy after biliary drainage in hilar bile duct cancer. Arch Surg 1995;130(7): 759–63.
38. Miyagawa S, Makuuchi M, Kawasaki S, et al. Outcome of major hepatectomy with pancreatoduodenectomy for advanced biliary malignancies. World J Surg 1996;20(1):77–80.
39. Seyama Y, Makuuchi M. Current surgical treatment for bile duct cancer. World J Gastroenterol 2007;13(10):1505–15.
40. Yamaguchi K, Chijiiwa K, Saiki S, et al. Carcinoma of the extrahepatic bile duct: mode of spread and its prognostic implications. Hepatogastroenterology 1997; 44(17):1256–61.

41. Sakamoto E, Nimura Y, Hayakawa N, et al. The pattern of infiltration at the proximal border of hilar bile duct carcinoma: a histologic analysis of 62 resected cases. Ann Surg 1998;227(3):405–11.
42. Ebata T, Watanabe H, Ajioka Y, et al. Pathological appraisal of lines of resection for bile duct carcinoma. Br J Surg 2002;89(10):1260–7.
43. Ogura Y, Takahashi K, Tabata M, et al. Clinicopathological study on carcinoma of the extrahepatic bile duct with special focus on cancer invasion on the surgical margins. World J Surg 1994;18(5):778–84.
44. Sarmiento JM, Nagorney DM. Hepatic resection in the treatment of perihilar cholangiocarcinoma. Surg Oncol Clin N Am 2002;11(4):893–908, viii–ix.
45. Clancy TE, Ashley SW. Pancreaticoduodenectomy (Whipple operation). Surg Oncol Clin N Am 2005;14(3):533–52, vii.
46. Kennedy EP, Yeo CJ. Pancreaticoduodenectomy with extended retroperitoneal lymphadenectomy for periampullary adenocarcinoma. Surg Oncol Clin N Am 2007;16(1):157–76.
47. Mizumoto R, Kawarada Y, Yamawaki T, et al. Resectability and functional reserve of the liver with obstructive jaundice in dogs. Am J Surg 1979;137(6):768–72.
48. Hatfield AR, Tobias R, Terblanche J, et al. Preoperative external biliary drainage in obstructive jaundice. A prospective controlled clinical trial. Lancet 1982; 2(8304):896–9.
49. Blamey SL, Fearon KC, Gilmour WH, et al. Prediction of risk in biliary surgery. Br J Surg 1983;70(9):535–8.
50. Gundry SR, Strodel WE, Knol JA, et al. Efficacy of preoperative biliary tract decompression in patients with obstructive jaundice. Arch Surg 1984;119(6): 703–8.
51. Pitt HA, Gomes AS, Lois JF, et al. Does preoperative percutaneous biliary drainage reduce operative risk or increase hospital cost? Ann Surg 1985; 201(5):545–53.
52. Lai EC, Mok FP, Fan ST, et al. Preoperative endoscopic drainage for malignant obstructive jaundice. Br J Surg 1994;81(8):1195–8.
53. Kawarada Y, Higashiguchi T, Yokoi H, et al. Preoperative biliary drainage in obstructive jaundice. Hepatogastroenterology 1995;42(4):300–7.
54. Nakeeb A, Pitt HA. The role of preoperative biliary decompression in obstructive jaundice. Hepatogastroenterology 1995;42(4):332–7.
55. Sewnath ME, Karsten TM, Prins MH, et al. A meta-analysis on the efficacy of preoperative biliary drainage for tumors causing obstructive jaundice. Ann Surg 2002;236(1):17–27.
56. Povoski SP, Karpeh MS Jr, Conlon KC, et al. Association of preoperative biliary drainage with postoperative outcome following pancreaticoduodenectomy. Ann Surg 1999;230(2):131–42.
57. Sewnath ME, Birjmohun RS, Rauws EA, et al. The effect of preoperative biliary drainage on postoperative complications after pancreaticoduodenectomy. J Am Coll Surg 2001;192(6):726–34.
58. Sakata J, Shirai Y, Wakai T, et al. Catheter tract implantation metastases associated with percutaneous biliary drainage for extrahepatic cholangiocarcinoma. World J Gastroenterol 2005;11(44):7024–7.
59. Belghiti J, Hiramatsu K, Benoist S, et al. Seven hundred forty-seven hepatectomies in the 1990s: an update to evaluate the actual risk of liver resection. J Am Coll Surg 2000;191(1):38–46.
60. Ogura Y, Kawarada Y. Surgical strategies for carcinoma of the hepatic duct confluence. Br J Surg 1998;85(1):20–4.

61. Kondo S, Hirano S, Ambo Y, et al. Forty consecutive resections of hilar cholangiocarcinoma with no postoperative mortality and no positive ductal margins: results of a prospective study. Ann Surg 2004;240(1):95–101.
62. Liu CL, Fan ST, Lo CM, et al. Improved operative and survival outcomes of surgical treatment for hilar cholangiocarcinoma. Br J Surg 2006;93(12):1488–94.
63. Cherqui D, Benoist S, Malassagne B, et al. Major liver resection for carcinoma in jaundiced patients without preoperative biliary drainage. Arch Surg 2000;135(3): 302–8.
64. Kamiya S, Nagino M, Kanazawa H, et al. The value of bile replacement during external biliary drainage: an analysis of intestinal permeability, integrity, and microflora. Ann Surg 2004;239(4):510–7.
65. Hochwald SN, Burke EC, Jarnagin WR, et al. Association of preoperative biliary stenting with increased postoperative infectious complications in proximal cholangiocarcinoma. Arch Surg 1999;134(3):261–6.
66. Jagannath P, Dhir V, Shrikhande S, et al. Effect of preoperative biliary stenting on immediate outcome after pancreaticoduodenectomy. Br J Surg 2005;92(3): 356–61.
67. Cortes A, Sauvanet A, Bert F, et al. Effect of bile contamination on immediate outcomes after pancreaticoduodenectomy for tumor. J Am Coll Surg 2006; 202(1):93–9.
68. Noie T, Sugawara Y, Imamura H, et al. Selective versus total drainage for biliary obstruction in the hepatic hilus: an experimental study. Surgery 2001;130(1): 74–81.
69. Ishizawa T, Hasegawa K, Sano K, et al. Selective versus total biliary drainage for obstructive jaundice caused by a hepatobiliary malignancy. Am J Surg 2007; 193(2):149–54.
70. Neuhaus P, Jonas S, Bechstein WO, et al. Extended resections for hilar cholangiocarcinoma. Ann Surg 1999;230(6):808–18 [discussion: 819].
71. Watanapa P. Recovery patterns of liver function after complete and partial surgical biliary decompression. Am J Surg 1996;171(2):230–4.
72. Liu CL, Lo CM, Lai EC, et al. Endoscopic retrograde cholangiopancreatography and endoscopic endoprosthesis insertion in patients with Klatskin tumors. Arch Surg 1998;133(3):293–6.
73. Rerknimitr R, Kladcharoen N, Mahachai V, et al. Result of endoscopic biliary drainage in hilar cholangiocarcinoma. J Clin Gastroenterol 2004;38(6):518–23.
74. Mansfield SD, Barakat O, Charnley RM, et al. Management of hilar cholangiocarcinoma in the North of England: pathology, treatment, and outcome. World J Gastroenterol 2005;11(48):7625–30.
75. Makuuchi M, Takayasu K, Takuma T, et al. Preoperative transcatheter embolization of the portal venous branch for patients receiving extended lobectomy due to teh bile duct carcinoma. J Jpn Surg Assoc 1984;45:1558–64.
76. Makuuchi M, Thai BL, Takayasu K, et al. Preoperative portal embolization to increase safety of major hepatectomy for hilar bile duct carcinoma: a preliminary report. Surgery 1990;107(5):521–7.
77. Abulkhir A, Limongelli P, Healey AJ, et al. Preoperative portal vein embolization for major liver resection: a meta-analysis. Ann Surg 2008;247(1):49–57.
78. Kubota K, Makuuchi M, Kusaka K, et al. Measurement of liver volume and hepatic functional reserve as a guide to decision-making in resectional surgery for hepatic tumors. Hepatology 1997;26(5):1176–81.
79. Clavien PA, Petrowsky H, DeOliveira ML, et al. Strategies for safer liver surgery and partial liver transplantation. N Engl J Med 2007;356(15):1545–59.

80. Ribero D, Abdalla EK, Madoff DC, et al. Portal vein embolization before major hepatectomy and its effects on regeneration, resectability and outcome. Br J Surg 2007;94(11):1386–94.
81. Seyama Y, Kokudo N. Assessment of liver fucntion for safe hepatic resection. Hepatol Res 2009;39:107–16.
82. Launois B, Terblanche J, Lakehal M, et al. Proximal bile duct cancer: high resectability rate and 5-year survival. Ann Surg 1999;230(2):266–75.
83. Mizumoto R, Suzuki H. Surgical anatomy of the hepatic hilum with special reference to the caudate lobe. World J Surg 1988;12(1):2–10.
84. Ogura Y, Mizumoto R, Tabata M, et al. Surgical treatment of carcinoma of the hepatic duct confluence: analysis of 55 resected carcinomas. World J Surg 1993;17(1):85–92 [discussion: 92–3].
85. Kogure K, Kuwano H, Fujimaki N, et al. Relation among portal segmentation, proper hepatic vein, and external notch of the caudate lobe in the human liver. Ann Surg 2000;231(2):223–8.
86. Suzuki M, Takahashi T, Ouchi K, et al. The development and extension of hepatohilar bile duct carcinoma. A three-dimensional tumor mapping in the intrahepatic biliary tree visualized with the aid of a graphics computer system. Cancer 1989;64(3):658–66.
87. Nimura Y, Hayakawa N, Kamiya J, et al. Hepatic segmentectomy with caudate lobe resection for bile duct carcinoma of the hepatic hilus. World J Surg 1990; 14(4):535–43 [discussion: 544].
88. Sugiura Y, Nakamura S, Iida S, et al. Extensive resection of the bile ducts combined with liver resection for cancer of the main hepatic duct junction: a cooperative study of the Keio Bile Duct Cancer Study Group. Surgery 1994; 115(4):445–51.
89. Tashiro S, Tsuji T, Kanemitsu K, et al. Prolongation of survival for carcinoma at the hepatic duct confluence. Surgery 1993;113(3):270–8.
90. Tsao JI, Nimura Y, Kamiya J, et al. Management of hilar cholangiocarcinoma: comparison of an American and a Japanese experience. Ann Surg 2000; 232(2):166–74.
91. Pichlmayr R, Weimann A, Klempnauer J, et al. Surgical treatment in proximal bile duct cancer. A single-center experience. Ann Surg 1996;224(5):628–38.
92. Kosuge T, Yamamoto J, Shimada K, et al. Improved surgical results for hilar cholangiocarcinoma with procedures including major hepatic resection. Ann Surg 1999;230(5):663–71.
93. Yamanaka N, Yasui C, Yamanaka J, et al. Left hemihepatectomy with microsurgical reconstruction of the right-sided hepatic vasculature. A strategy for preserving hepatic function in patients with proximal bile duct cancer. Langenbecks Arch Surg 2001;386(5):364–8.
94. Nagino M, Nimura Y, Kamiya J, et al. Right or left trisegment portal vein embolization before hepatic trisegmentectomy for hilar bile duct carcinoma. Surgery 1995;117(6):677–81.
95. Noie T, Bandai Y, Kubota K, et al. Extended right trisegmentectomy for hilar bile duct carcinoma. Hepatogastroenterology 1997;44(16):998–1001.
96. Nagino M, Kamiya J, Kanai M, et al. Right trisegment portal vein embolization for biliary tract carcinoma: technique and clinical utility. Surgery 2000;127(2): 155–60.
97. Shimada K, Sano T, Sakamoto Y, et al. Safety and effectiveness of left hepatic trisegmentectomy for hilar cholangiocarcinoma. World J Surg 2005;29(6): 723–7.

98. Nagino M, Kamiya J, Arai T, et al. "Anatomic" right hepatic trisectionectomy (extended right hepatectomy) with caudate lobectomy for hilar cholangiocarcinoma. Ann Surg 2006;243(1):28–32.

99. Nimura Y, Hayakawa N, Kamiya J, et al. Hepatopancreatoduodenectomy for advanced carcinoma of the biliary tract. Hepatogastroenterology 1991;38(2): 170–5.

100. Miwa S, Kobayashi A, Akahane Y, et al. Is major hepatectomy with pancreatoduodenectomy justified for advanced biliary malignancy? J Hepatobiliary Pancreat Surg 2007;14(2):136–41.

101. Hirono S, Tani M, Kawai M, et al. Indication of hepatopancreatoduodenectomy for biliary tract cancer. World J Surg 2006;30(4):567–73 [discussion: 574–5].

102. Ebata T, Nagino M, Nishio H, et al. Right hepatopancreatoduodenectomy: improvements over 23 years to attain acceptability. J Hepatobiliary Pancreat Surg 2007;14(2):131–5.

103. Wakai T, Shirai Y, Tsuchiya Y, et al. Combined major hepatectomy and pancreaticoduodenectomy for locally advanced biliary carcinoma: long-term results. World J Surg 2008;32(6):1067–74.

104. Mimura H, Kim H, Ochiai Y, et al. Radical block resection of hepatoduodenal ligament for carcinoma of the bile duct with double catheter bypass for portal circulation. Surg Gynecol Obstet 1988;167(6):527–9.

105. Miyagawa S, Makuuchi M, Kawasaki S, et al. Second-stage pancreatojejunostomy following pancreatoduodenectomy in high-risk patients. Am J Surg 1994;168(1):66–8.

106. Seyama Y, Kubota K, Kobayashi T, et al. Two-staged pancreatoduodenectomy with external drainage of pancreatic juice and omental graft technique. J Am Coll Surg 1998;187(1):103–5.

107. Kubota K, Makuuchi M, Takayama T, et al. Appraisal of two-staged pancreatoduodenectomy: its technical aspects and outcome. Hepatogastroenterology 2000;47(31):269–74.

108. Hasegawa K, Kokudo N, Sano K, et al. Two-stage pancreatojejunostomy in pancreaticoduodenectomy: a retrospective analysis of short-term results. Am J Surg 2008;196(1):3–10.

109. Nimura Y, Hayakawa N, Kamiya J, et al. Combined portal vein and liver resection for carcinoma of the biliary tract. Br J Surg 1991;78(6):727–31.

110. Gerhards MF, van Gulik TM, de Wit LT, et al. Evaluation of morbidity and mortality after resection for hilar cholangiocarcinoma–a single center experience. Surgery 2000;127(4):395–404.

111. Wakai T, Shirai Y, Moroda T, et al. Impact of ductal resection margin status on long-term survival in patients undergoing resection for extrahepatic cholangiocarcinoma. Cancer 2005;103(6):1210–6.

112. Hwang S, Lee SG, Kim KH, et al. Extended extrahepatic bile duct resection to avoid performing pancreatoduodenectomy in patients with mid bile duct cancer. Dig Surg 2008;25(1):74–9.

113. Di Carlo V, Zerbi A, Balzano G, et al. Pylorus-preserving pancreaticoduodenectomy versus conventional whipple operation. World J Surg 1999;23(9):920–5.

114. Seiler CA, Wagner M, Sadowski C, et al. Randomized prospective trial of pylorus-preserving vs. classic duodenopancreatectomy (Whipple procedure): initial clinical results. J Gastrointest Surg 2000;4(5):443–52.

115. Tran KT, Smeenk HG, van Eijck CH, et al. Pylorus preserving pancreaticoduodenectomy versus standard Whipple procedure: a prospective, randomized,

multicenter analysis of 170 patients with pancreatic and periampullary tumors. Ann Surg 2004;240(5):738–45.

116. Seiler CA, Wagner M, Bachmann T, et al. Randomized clinical trial of pylorus-preserving duodenopancreatectomy versus classical Whipple resection-long term results. Br J Surg 2005;92(5):547–56.

117. Diener MK, Knaebel HP, Heukaufer C, et al. A systematic review and meta-analysis of pylorus-preserving versus classical pancreaticoduodenectomy for surgical treatment of periampullary and pancreatic carcinoma. Ann Surg 2007;245(2):187–200.

118. Roder JD, Stein HJ, Siewert JR. Carcinoma of the periampullary region: who benefits from portal vein resection? Am J Surg 1996;171(1):170–4 [discussion: 174–5].

119. Yeo CJ, Sohn TA, Cameron JL, et al. Periampullary adenocarcinoma: analysis of 5-year survivors. Ann Surg 1998;227(6):821–31.

120. Riall TS, Cameron JL, Lillemoe KD, et al. Pancreaticoduodenectomy with or without distal gastrectomy and extended retroperitoneal lymphadenectomy for periampullary adenocarcinoma–part 3: update on 5-year survival. J Gastrointest Surg 2005;9(9):1191–204 [discussion: 1204–6].

121. Nelson H, Petrelli N, Carlin A, et al. Guidelines 2000 for colon and rectal cancer surgery. J Natl Cancer Inst 2001;93(8):583–96.

122. Tepper JE, O'Connell MJ, Niedzwiecki D, et al. Impact of number of nodes retrieved on outcome in patients with rectal cancer. J Clin Oncol 2001;19(1): 157–63.

123. Le Voyer TE, Sigurdson ER, Hanlon AL, et al. Colon cancer survival is associated with increasing number of lymph nodes analyzed: a secondary survey of intergroup trial INT-0089. J Clin Oncol 2003;21(15):2912–9.

124. Smith DD, Schwarz RR, Schwarz RE. Impact of total lymph node count on staging and survival after gastrectomy for gastric cancer: data from a large US-population database. J Clin Oncol 2005;23(28):7114–24.

125. Pawlik TM, Gleisner AL, Cameron JL, et al. Prognostic relevance of lymph node ratio following pancreaticoduodenectomy for pancreatic cancer. Surgery 2007; 141(5):610–8.

126. Tomlinson JS, Jain S, Bentrem DJ, et al. Accuracy of staging node-negative pancreas cancer: a potential quality measure. Arch Surg 2007;142(8):767–74 [discussion: 773–4].

127. Sobin LH, Wittekind C, editors. International Union Against Cancer, TNM classification of malignant tumors. 6th edition. New York: Wiley-Liss; 2002.

128. Murakami Y, Uemura K, Hayashidani Y, et al. Prognostic significance of lymph node metastasis and surgical margin status for distal cholangiocarcinoma. J Surg Oncol 2007;95(3):207–12.

129. Klempnauer J, Ridder GJ, von Wasielewski R, et al. Resectional surgery of hilar cholangiocarcinoma: a multivariate analysis of prognostic factors. J Clin Oncol 1997;15(3):947–54.

130. Miyazaki M, Ito H, Nakagawa K, et al. Parenchyma-preserving hepatectomy in the surgical treatment of hilar cholangiocarcinoma. J Am Coll Surg 1999; 189(6):575–83.

Indications for Neoadjuvant, Adjuvant, and Palliative Chemotherapy in the Treatment of Biliary Tract Cancers

Fidel David Huitzil-Melendez, MD[a], Eileen M. O'Reilly, MD[a,b],
Austin Duffy, MD[a], Ghassan K. Abou-Alfa, MD[a,b],*

KEYWORDS

- Biliary tract cancers • Cholangiocarcinoma
- Gallbladder cancer • Chemotherapy
- Regional chemotherapy • Targeted agents
- Adjuvant therapy

Carcinomas arising from the biliary tree epithelium are uncommon malignancies in the United States. According to the Surveillance, Epidemiology and End Results program, gallbladder cancer is the most common biliary tract malignancy, with an age-adjusted incidence of 1.2184 cases per 100,000 in 2005.[1] The incidence of intrahepatic cholangiocarcinoma is lower, but has increased in recent years from 0.13 cases per 100,000 in 1973 to 0.67 cases per 100,000 in 1997.[2] In 2008, 9520 new cases of gallbladder and other bile duct cancers were estimated to occur in the United States. In addition, 21,370 new cases of primary liver cancer, of which approximately 10% are intrahepatic cholangiocarcinomas, were also estimated for 2008.[3]

According to Surveillance, Epidemiology and End Results, the estimated overall 5-year survival rate in year 2000 for gallbladder cancer was 16.65% and that of liver and intrahepatic bile duct cancer was only 11.82%.[1] The poor prognosis is in part explained by advanced disease at presentation in most cases. Only 31% of patients with gallbladder cancer and 36% of patients with liver and bile duct cancer have localized disease at presentation.[1] Even surgically treated patients experience high rates of recurrent disease.[4–6] In this context, it is clear that effective adjuvant treatment strategies are desperately needed for successfully resected patients and that most

[a] Section of Gastrointestinal Oncology, Memorial Sloan-Kettering Cancer Center, 1275 York Avenue, New York, NY 10022, USA
[b] Weill Medical College at Cornell University, New York, NY, USA
* Corresponding author.
E-mail address: abou-alg@mskcc.org (G.K. Abou-Alfa).

Surg Oncol Clin N Am 18 (2009) 361–379
doi:10.1016/j.soc.2008.12.006
1055-3207/08/$ – see front matter © 2009 Elsevier Inc. All rights reserved.

surgonc.theclinics.com

patients with biliary tract cancers are candidates for palliative therapy at some point in the course of their disease.

This article reviews the available evidence to support indications of systemic chemotherapy in the palliative and perioperative settings.

SYSTEMIC CHEMOTHERAPY IN ADVANCED DISEASE
Meta-Analysis

Many chemotherapy agents and regimens have been tested in patients with advanced biliary tract cancers. The most comprehensive evaluation of the activity of systemic chemotherapy in advanced biliary tract cancers derives from a pooled analysis of 104 chemotherapy trials published in English from 1985 to 2006, comprising 112 trial arms and 2810 patients.[7] Several aspects of available clinical trials of systemic chemotherapy in advanced biliary tract cancers must be highlighted. Despite evidence that gallbladder, intrahepatic, and extrahepatic bile duct carcinomas differ not only in risk factors and clinical manifestations but also in molecular pathogenesis and prognosis,[8] clinical trials evaluating the activity of systemic therapies often pool these carcinomas under the common denomination of advanced biliary tract carcinomas. As such, possible distinct responses to systemic therapies cannot be discerned with confidence. Most are single-arm phase II trials. Only one phase III trial and two randomized phase II trials were identified in this meta-analysis. Only a minority of the trials reported statistical considerations, such as sample size calculation, null and alternative hypothesis, significance level, and power. The mean number of patients per trial was 25.1 (range, 5–65). Results from well-designed controlled trials evaluating the activity of systemic chemotherapy in advanced biliary tract cancers are lacking, and important questions, such as whether chemotherapy improves survival over best supportive care, whether combination chemotherapy is superior to single-agent therapy in terms of survival, and which is the reference regimen in this disease, remain without a solid evidence-based answer.

Nonetheless, the pooled analysis has defined relevant outcomes for chemotherapy in advanced biliary tract cancers. Response rate defined as complete response and partial response and tumor control rate defined as complete response, partial response, and stable disease showed a weak ($r = 0.2$ and $r = 0.26$, respectively) but significant correlation with time to tumor progression and overall survival. Time to tumor progression showed a strong ($r = 0.73$) and statistically significant ($P = .000$) correlation with overall survival. Although comparisons among regimens evaluated in single-arm phase II trials are not appropriate, the results of the pooled analysis may be the best evidence available regarding the activity of systemic chemotherapy in advanced biliary tract cancers and may define chemotherapy historical controls useful for the design of future clinical trials.

Results of the pooled analysis are summarized in **Table 1**. The pooled response rate was 22.6% (95% confidence interval [CI], 21–24.2; N = 2810) and the pooled tumor control rate was 57.3% (95% CI, 55.3–59.3; N = 2386). Median time to progression was 4.1 months (1543 patients) and median overall survival was 8.2 months (2197 patients). A regression equation showed that a 10% increment in response corresponded to an 8% increase of tumor control rate, a 0.7-month increase of time to progression, and a 0.6-month increase of overall survival. A 1-month increase in time to progression corresponded to a 1.3-month increase of overall survival.

Reliable comparisons among chemotherapy regimens can only be derived from well-designed and well-conducted randomized controlled trials that minimize a myriad of potential biases, including selection bias. Comparisons derived from the pooled

Table 1
Activity of different chemotherapy regimens in advanced biliary tract carcinomas

	N	RR%	TCR%	TTP (mon)	OS (mon)
Fluoropyrimidines	1428	22	58	—	—
Gemcitabine	1369	26	61	4.6 versus 3.7	—
Platinum compounds	1123	30	62	NS	NS
Anthracyclines	247	17	58	—	—
Mitomycin C	162	17.5	61	—	—
Taxanes	99	9	45	—	—
Irinotecan	144	14.5	44	—	—
All patients	2810	22.6	57.3	4.1	8.2

Subgroups were defined by regimens containing a particular drug, and were compared with all other patients treated with regimens that did not contain that particular drug, regardless of other drugs.

Data from Eckel F, Schmid RM. Chemotherapy in advanced biliary tract carcinoma: a pooled analysis of clinical trials. Br J Cancer 2007;96:896–902.

analysis must be interpreted with caution. Two-drug regimens (N = 1499) compared with monotherapy regimens (N = 971) showed superior response rates (28% versus 15.3%; P = .000); tumor control rates (61% versus 50.4%; P = .000); median time to progression (4.4 versus 3.4 months; P = .015); and a trend toward improved median overall survival (9.3 versus 7.5 months; P = .061). Three or more drug regimens (N = 340) compared with two drug regimens (N = 1499) resulted in lower response rate (19.1% versus 28%; P = .000) with no difference in median overall survival (9 versus 9.3 months). Regimens that included gemcitabine or cisplatin compared with regimens that did not include these drugs consistently resulted in statistically significant higher response rate (P = .000) and tumor control rate (P = .000). Further subgroup analyses focused on combinations of fluoropyrimidine, gemcitabine, and cisplatin and revealed that the addition of platinum compounds to fluoropyrimidine resulted in an 8.7% increase in response rate, whereas the addition of platinum compounds to gemcitabine resulted in a 17% improvement.

A number of trials included gallbladder cancer only (N = 500) or cholangiocarcinoma only (N = 471) patients. Although the response rate seemed higher in trials including gallbladder cancer only patients compared with trials including cholangiocarcinoma only patients (34.4% versus 20.2%; P = .000), median overall survival was significantly better in trials of patients with cholangiocarcinoma compared with gallbladder cancer (9.3 versus 7.2 months; P = .048).

Randomized Trials in Advanced Disease

To determine if chemotherapy improves tumor symptom control, quality of life, and overall survival, 93 patients with advanced pancreatic adenocarcinoma and biliary tract cancers were included in a randomized control trial comparing chemotherapy with best supportive care.[9] Chemotherapy consisted of 5-fluorouracil, 500 mg/m^2 bolus intravenously (IV), followed by leucovorin, 60 mg/m^2 on 2 consecutive days, every 2 weeks. Younger patients with better performance status received the same regimen for 3 consecutive days plus etoposide, 120 mg/m^2 for 3 consecutive days. Patients randomized to best supportive care were allowed to receive chemotherapy if best supportive care did not control symptoms. Overall survival (6 versus 2.5 months; P<.01), symptom control (43% versus 12%), and average quality-adjusted survival

(4 versus 1 month) were all improved in patients in the chemotherapy arm. When only biliary tract cancers patients were analyzed (N = 37), the overall survival improvement was maintained in favor of the chemotherapy arm (6.5 versus 2.5 months).

Two other randomized trials compared single-agent chemotherapy with two-drug regimens (**Table 2**). The benefit of adding cisplatin to 5-fluorouracil was examined in a randomized phase II trial that included 58 patients with biliary tract cancers.[10] Patients randomized to the single-agent arm were treated with 7-week cycles of weekly high-dose 5-fluorouracil at 3 g/m^2 24-hour infusion for 6 weeks followed by 1 week rest. Patients randomized to the combination arm received 7-week cycles of weekly infusions of leucovorin, 500 mg/m^2, followed by 5-fluorouracil, 2 g/m^2, 24-hour infusion for 6 weeks followed by 1 week rest, and cisplatin, 50 mg/m^2, every 2 weeks for 6 weeks, followed by 1 week rest. Treatment arms did not seem to be different in terms of efficacy. Response rate was 7.1 (95% CI, 0.9–23.5) in the single-agent arm and 18.5% (95% CI, 6.3–38.1) in the combination arm; median progression-free survival was 3.3 months in both arms and median overall survival was 5 months (95% CI, 4–7.4) in the single-agent arm and 8 months (95% CI, 5.8–11.8) in the combination arm. Grade 3 and 4 toxicities were higher in the combination arm, however, specifically neutropenia (4% versus 26%); anemia (0% versus 11%); thrombocytopenia (0% versus 7%); diarrhea (0% versus 11%); vomiting (7% versus 14%); and mucositis (0% versus 4%). The authors concluded that given the increased occurrence of severe side effects in the combination arm in the setting of patients with a poor life expectancy, evaluation of the combination of 5-fluorouracil and cisplatin in a phase III trial could not be recommended.

Another randomized phase II trial examined the benefit of adding cisplatin to single-agent gemcitabine for the treatment of patients with biliary tract cancers.[11] Eighty-six patients were randomized to receive either single-agent gemcitabine alone or the combination of gemcitabine and cisplatin. Single-agent gemcitabine was given at 1000 mg/m^2 on days 1, 8, and 15 every 28 days for six cycles (24 weeks). The combination arm consisted of gemcitabine at 1000 mg/m^2 and cisplatin at 25 mg/m^2 on days 1 and 8 of an every 3-week cycle, for eight cycles (24 weeks). Primary end point, 6-month progression-free survival was 57.1% for the combination arm and 47.7% for the single-agent arm. Median time to progression was 8 months for gemcitabine and cisplatin versus 4 months for gemcitabine alone. Tumor control rate increased from 57.6% for single-agent gemcitabine to 75.7% for the combination. This improved activity was at the expense of increased lethargy in the combination arm (28.6% versus 9.1%). Other toxicities seemed to occur with similar incidence. Grade 3 and 4 toxicities for 42 patients treated in the combination arm included anemia 2.4%, leucopenia 4.8%, neutropenia 14.3%, thrombocytopenia 11.9%, lethargy 28.6%, nausea and vomiting 4.8%, anorexia 4.8%, neutropenic sepsis 2.4%, and nonneutropenic sepsis 19%. Grade 3 and 4 toxicities for 44 patients treated with single-agent gemcitabine included anemia 4.5%, leucopenia 6.8%, thrombocytopenia 9.1%, anorexia 2.3%, and nonneutropenic sepsis 18.2%, with no cases of neutropenic sepsis reported. The authors did not attempt any statistical analysis given limitation of sample size. Instead, they redesigned their study to a randomized phase III study powered to detect survival differences. This study is still underway and accruing patients (ABC-02 study).

Another two randomized trials compared the activity of combination chemotherapy regimens. These trials were designed under the assumption that combination therapy would lead to better outcome compared with single-agent chemotherapy. Fifty-one patients with advanced biliary tract cancers were enrolled in a randomized phase II trial and were randomly allocated to treatment with mitomycin-C, 8 mg/m^2 on day 1, plus gemcitabine, 2000 mg/m^2 on days 1 and 15 every 4 weeks, or mitomycin-C, 8 mg/m^2

on day 1, plus capecitabine, 2000 mg/m^2/d on days 1 to 14, every 4 weeks.[12] Chemotherapy was continued until progression of disease or until 6 months of therapy were completed. In terms of efficacy, the gemcitabine arm response rates were partial response 20% and stable disease 36%. Median progression-free survival was 4.2 months and median overall survival was 6.7 months. For the capecitabine-based arm, response rates were partial response 31% and stable disease 34.5%. Median progression-free survival was 5.35 months and median overall survival was 9.25 months. The 1-year survival rate was 23% in the gemcitabine arm and 41% in the capecitabine arm. Grade 3 neutropenia and thrombocytopenia was observed in 13% of patients in the gemcitabine group and 17% of the patients in the capecitabine group. These represented the most frequent serious toxicities. The authors concluded that both regimens had acceptable level of antitumor activity and were well tolerated and recommended further evaluation of the mitomycin-C and capecitabine combination.

The combination of 5-flurouracil, etoposide, and leucovorin (FELV) was compared with the combination of epirubicin, cisplatin, and infusional 5-flurouracil (ECF) in a randomized phase III trial.[13] The FELV regimen consisted of 5-flurouracil, 600 mg/m^2 IV bolus on days 1 to 3, etoposide, 120 mg/m^2 40-minute IV infusion on days 1 to 3, and leucovorin, 60 mg/m^2 IV bolus on days 1 to 3, every 3 weeks. The ECF regimen consisted of 5-flurouracil, 200 mg/m^2 continuous infusion for 24 weeks, epirubicin, 50 mg/m^2 on day 1, and cisplatin, 60 mg/m^2 on day 1, every 3 weeks. The trial accrued only 54 patients in 6 years and was closed. In terms of efficacy, patients assigned to FELV experienced a partial response of 15% and stable disease of 45%. Symptom control was reported as follows: pain 78%, weight loss 78%, nausea 75%, anorexia 64%, and lethargy 20%. Median survival was close to 1 year (367 days). Patients treated on the ECF arm experienced complete response 3.8%, partial response 15.4%, and stable disease 46.2%. Rates of symptom resolution were anorexia 92%, weight loss 82%, pain 80%, nausea 67%, and lethargy 43%. Median overall survival was close to 9 months (275 days). The survival difference between the two treatment arms was not statistically significant ($P = .2059$). In terms of hematologic toxicity profile, FELV was associated with grade 3 and 4 anemia 11.5%, neutropenia 53.8%, and thrombocytopenia 8.3%. ECF was associated with grade 3 and 4 anemia 25.9%, neutropenia 25.9%, and thrombocytopenia 3.7%. Grade 3 and 4 nonhematologic toxicities in the FELV arm were alopecia 75%, lethargy 58.3%, infection 41.7%, diarrhea 12.5%, nausea and vomiting 8.3%, stomatitis 8.3%, fever 8.3%, and neutropenic fever 4.2%. Grade 3 and 4 nonhematologic toxicity in the ECF arm were lethargy 56%, alopecia 40%, infection 16%, nausea and vomiting 16%, diarrhea 12%, fever 12%, and stomatitis 8%. Authors concluded that chemotherapy can provide good symptom control in this disease and seems to prolong overall survival. The study was considered underpowered to select a reference regimen.

5-Flurouracil and Platinum Combinations

A phase II study (**Table 3**) included 25 previously untreated patients with inoperable locally advanced (N = 3) or metastatic (N = 22) biliary tract cancer.[14] Eleven patients had gallbladder cancer and 14 patients had intrahepatic or extrahepatic cholangiocarcinoma. The chemotherapy regimen consisted of 5-flurouracil at 1 g/m^2/d in continuous IV infusion for 5 consecutive days and cisplatin at 100 mg/m^2/d on day 2 in a 1-hour infusion with standard hyperhydration. The overall response rate was 24%, the median survival was 10 months, and the 1-year survival rate was 33%. Grade 3 toxicities included neutropenia (six patients, 24%); nausea and vomiting (six patients, 24%); thrombocytopenia (two patients, 8%); leucopenia (4%); stomatitis

Table 2
Randomized trials in patients with advanced biliary tract carcinomas

Author	N	Group A	Group B	Outcome	Comments
Glimelius et al	37	5-FU, 500 mg/m^2 × 2–3 d LV, 60 mg/m^2 × 2–3 d ± Etoposide, 120 mg/m^2 × 2–3 d Every 2 wk (younger patients and with better performance status received etoposide)	Best supportive care	OS A: 6 mon B: 2.5 mon	Subgroup analysis from 93 randomized patients with pancreatobiliary malignancies. Best supportive care group allowed to receive chemotherapy if best supportive care did not control symptoms.
Ducreaux et al	58	LV, 500 mg/m2 weekly × 6 5-FU, 2 g/m2 24-h infusion × 6 Cisplatin, 50 mg/m2 every 2 wk × 3 Every 7 wk	5-FU 3 g/m2 24-h infusion weekly × 6 Every 7 wk	Partial response: A: 18.5% B: 7.1% PFS: A: 3.3 mon B: 3.3 mon OS: A: 8 mon B: 5 mon	Randomized phase II. Increased toxicity in the combination therapy arm.
Valle et al	86	Gemcitabine, 1000 mg/m2 weekly × 2 Cisplatin, 25 mg/m2 weekly × 2 Every 3 wk for 8 cycles	Gemcitabine, 1000 mg/m^2 weekly × 3 for 6 cycles	6-mon PFS A: 57.1% B: 47.1% TTP: A: 8 mon B: 4 mon TCR: A: 75.7% B: 57.6%	Randomized phase II. Redesigned into phase III with OS and quality of life end points.

Kornek et al	2004	Mitomycin C, 8 mg/m2 d 1 Gemcitabine, 2000 mg/m2 d 1 and 15 Every 4 wk	Mitomycin C, 8 mg/m2 d 1 Capecitabine, 2000 mg/m2/d d 1–14 Every 4 wk	Partial response: A: 20% B: 31% PFS: A: 4.2 mon B: 5.3 mon OS A: 6.7 mon B: 9.5 mon	Randomized phase II. Group B recommended for further evaluation.
Rao et al	54	5-FU, 600 mg/m2 d 1–3 bolus Etoposide, 120 mg/m2 d 1–3 Leucovorin, 60 mg/m2 d 1–3	5-FU, 200 mg/m2/d continuous infusion 24 wk Epirubicin, 50 mg/m2 d 1 Cisplatin, 60 mg/m2 d 1 Every 3 wk	Partial response: A: 15% B: 19.2% OS A: 367 d B: 275 d	Randomized phase III closed because of slow accrual. Underpowered study to select a reference regimen. Both regimens resulted in good symptom control rate.

Abbreviations: 5-FU, 5-fluorouracil; LV, leucovorin; OS, overall survival; PFS, progression-free survival; TCR, tumor control rate; TTP, time to progression.

Table 3
Activity of fluoropyrimidine and platinum based chemotherapy regimens in advanced biliary tract carcinomas

Author	N	Fluoropyrimidine	Platinum Compound	Outcome	Comments
Ducreux et al	25	5-FU, 1 g/m2/d 24 h CI × 5 d Every 4 wk	Cisplatin, 100 mg/m2 d 2 Every 4 wk	PR: 24% OS: 10 mon 1-y survival: 33%	Febrile neutropenia: 16%
Taieb et al	29	LV, 200 mg/m2 2-h infusion × 2 d 5-FU, 400 mg/m2 bolus × 2 d 5-FU, 600 mg/m2 22-h infusion × 2 d Every 2 wk	Cisplatin, 50 mg/m2 d 2 Every 2 wk	PR: 34% OS: 9.5 mon	Improved therapeutic index. Documented symptomatic improvement.
Sanz-Altamira et al	14	LV, 25 mg/m2 × 4 d 5-FU, 400 mg/m2 × 4 d bolus Every 4 wk	Carboplatin, 300 mg/m2 d 1 Every 4 wk	PR: 21% OS: 5 mon	57% of patients had at least one episode of febrile neutropenia.
Nehls et al	16	LV, 500 mg/m2 2-h day 1 5-FU, 1.5-2 g/m2 22-h d 1 and 2 Every 2 wk	Oxaliplatin, 85 mg/m2 2-h d 1 Every 2 wk	PR: 19% TTP: 4.1 mon OS: 9.5 mon	Well tolerated. <2% grade 3 and 4 hematologic toxicity.
Lim et al	28	LV, 100 mg/m2 d 1 and 2 5-FU, 1000 mg/m2 24-h d 1 and 2 Every 3 wk	Oxaliplatin, 100 mg/m2 d 1 Every 3 wk	PR: 21.5% TTP: 3.5 mon OS: 10 mon	Grade 3 neutropenia 18% of patients.
Nehls et al	65	Capecitabine, 1000 mg/m2 twice a day d 1–14 Every 3 wk	Oxaliplatin, 130 mg/m2 d 1 Every 3 wk	Intrahepatic bile ducts: No PR TTP: 2.2 mon OS: 5.2 mon Extrahepatic bile ducts: RR: 25% TTP: 11.3 mon OS: 16.6 mon Gallbladder: RR: 30% TTP: 4.7 mon OS: 8 mon	Differential outcome according to site. Convenient schedule. Favorable toxicity profile.

Abbreviations: 5-FU, 5-fluorouracil; LV, leucovorin; OS, overall survival; PR, partial response; RR, response rate; TTP, time to progression.

(4%); and neurotoxicity (4%). Grade 4 side effects included neutropenia (4%); leuco-penia (8%); and thrombocytopenia (4%). Febrile neutropenia occurred in four patients (16%).

A more recent study by the same group suggests an improvement by adding leuco-vorin to the 5-fluorourcail and cisplatin combination, and modifying the chemotherapy schedule.[15] Twenty-nine patients with advanced or metastatic biliary tract cancer were prospectively evaluated. The treatment consisted of a biweekly administration of a 2-hour infusion of leucovorin, 200 mg/m^2, a 400 mg/m^2 bolus of 5-flurouracil, fol-lowed by a 22-hour continuous infusion of 600 mg/m^2 fluorouracil on 2 consecutive days and cisplatin, 50 mg/m^2 on day 2. The objective response rate was 34% and median overall survival was 9.5 months. Weight gain was observed in 45% of patients and performance status improved in 60%. Grade 3 toxicities included neutropenia 17%, nausea and vomiting 10%, anemia 7%, thrombocytopenia 7%, and neurotox-icity 3%. One patient had a grade 4 thrombocytopenia. There were no treatment-related deaths.

The combination of 5-fluorouracil and carboplatin has also been examined in this disease. A small phase II study included 14 consecutive patients with advanced unre-sectable gallbladder carcinoma (N = 4) or cholangiocarcinoma (N = 10).[16] Carboplatin was administered at 300 mg/m^2 IV on day 1 as a short infusion, leucovorin, 25 mg/m^2, with 5-fluorouracil, 400 mg/m^2 IV on days 1 to 4 as a bolus. Responses were only observed in 3 (21.4%) of 14 patients. The duration of responses were 8, 7+, and 26+ months for the three patients who responded. The dose-limiting toxicity was myelosuppression. Eight (57%) of the 14 patients had at least one episode of neutro-penia and fever. One patient required a platelet transfusion and three patients required transfusion for symptomatic anemia. Grade 3 mucositis occurred in three patients and grade 3 diarrhea occurred in one patient.

Infusional 5-fluorouracil and oxaliplatin (FOLFOX3) has been evaluated in a phase II trial that included 16 patients with advanced biliary tract cancer.[17] The site of the primary tumor was the gallbladder in seven patients, intrahepatic cholangiocarcinoma in seven patients, and extrahepatic cholangiocarcinoma in two patients. Patients were treated with oxaliplatin, 85 mg/m^2 over 2 hours, concurrent with leucovorin, 500 mg/m^2 on day 1, followed by continuous 5-fluorouracil infusion, 1.5 to 2 g/m^2 per 22 hours on days 1 and 2. Partial response was documented in 19% of the patients, whereas stable disease was observed in 37.5% of patients. Median time to progression was 4.1 months and median overall survival was 9.5 months. Toxic effects were reported on 146 courses. Both grade 4 adverse reactions (thrombocytopenia and nonfebrile leucopenia) and grade 3 adverse reactions (thrombocytopenia, mucositis, and infection) were observed in less than 2% of the cycles, respectively.

More recently, the combination of infusional 5-fluorouracil and oxaliplatin was tested in 28 patients with advanced biliary tract cancers of which 39% had progressed after first-line chemotherapy and 36% had an ECOG performance status of 2.[18] Oxaliplatin, 100 mg/m^2, was administered as a 2-hour IV infusion followed by leuco-vorin, 100 mg/m^2, as a bolus on day 1 followed by a 24-hour continuous infusion of 5-fluorouracil, 1000 mg/m^2 on days 1 and 2. Treatment was repeated every 3 weeks. One patient achieved a complete response and five patients achieved a partial response with an overall response rate of 21.5%. Nine patients showed stable disease (32.1%). Median time to progression was 3.5 months and median overall survival was 10 months. Grade 3 neutropenia was observed in 18% of patients, and six patients (21%) were given granulocyte colony-stimulating factor support. No cases of neutro-penic fever were reported. Other grade 3 and 4 toxicities included anemia (15%); thrombocytopenia (4%); nausea and vomiting in one patient; and neuropathy in another patient. Four patients developed grade 3 infection, two of them in the setting of biliary obstruction given progression of disease.

Capecitabine was substituted for infusional 5-fluorouracil in a recently reported phase II trial that evaluated 65 patients with advanced biliary tract cancer. Patients were treated with capecitabine, 1000 mg/m^2 per dose administered orally twice a day for 14 days, and oxaliplatin, 130 mg/m^2 administered as a 2-hour infusion on day 1, in an every 3-week cycle.[19] The primary site of disease was the gallbladder in 27 patients, the extrahepatic bile ducts in 20 patients, and the intrahepatic bile ducts in 18 patients. Efficacy was reported for gallbladder and extrahepatic bile ducts (group A) and intrahepatic bile ducts (group B) separately. Response rates for group A (N = 47) were as follows: 4% complete response, 23% partial response, and 49% stable disease. Median time to progression and median overall survival were 6.5 months (95% CI, 5.3–7.7 months) and 12.8 months (95% CI, 10.0–15.6 months), respectively. In group B (N = 18), responses were limited to 33% stable disease. Median time to progression and overall survival were 2.2 months (95% CI, 1.4–3.0 months) and 5.2 months (95% CI, 0.6–9.8 months), respectively. Differences in time to progression and overall survival were also observed between patients with extrahepatic cholangiocarcinoma and gallbladder cancer. Median time to progression was 11.3 months versus 4.7 months (P = .001). Median overall survival was 16.6 months versus 8 months, respectively (P = .03). Of note, 51% of the patients received second-line chemotherapy (single-agent gemcitabine, gemcitabine and capecitabine, mitomycin-C and gemcitabine).

Grade 3 toxicity in any cycle included thrombocytopenia 9%; nausea and vomiting 6%; diarrhea 5%; and hand-foot syndrome 5% (worst per patient). Grade 4 toxicity included infection 3%, neutropenia 2%, febrile neutropenia 2%, thrombocytopenia 2%, diarrhea 2%, and thromboembolic events 2%. In addition, grade 3 neuropathy was observed in 15% of patients and grade 4 in 2% of patients.

Gemcitabine and Platinum Combinations

Early reports evaluating a limited number of patients with advanced biliary tract cancer treated with the combination of gemcitabine and cisplatin (**Table 4**) showed an encouraging 50% and 64% response rate.[20,21] Larger confirmatory studies better defined the therapeutic potential of this combination. Thirty patients with advanced gallbladder cancer were included in a phase II trial and were treated with gemcitabine, 1000 mg/m^2 days 1 and 8, and cisplatin, 70 mg/m^2 day 1, on an every 3-week cycle for a maximum of six cycles.[22] Evaluation of response of 22 evaluable patients revealed 13.3% complete response, 23.3% partial response, and 23.3% stable disease. Median time to progression was 18 weeks and median overall survival was 20 weeks. Grade 3 toxicities included nausea and vomiting 27%, anemia 23%, neutropenia 17%, leucopenia 10%, thrombocytopenia 10%, hepatic 7%, renal 3%, and hemorrhagic 3%. Grade 4 toxicities included neutropenia 17%, anemia 13%, leucopenia 7%, thrombocytopenia 7%, hepatic 3%, renal 3%, and nausea and vomiting 3%.

A larger phase II study enrolled 43 patients with advanced biliary tract cancer and treated them with gemcitabine, 1250 mg/m^2 on a 30-minute IV infusion days 1 and 8, and cisplatin, 75 mg/m^2 in a 2-hour IV infusion day 1, every 3 weeks in the first-line setting.[23] The primary site was the intrahepatic bile ducts in 87.5% of 40 evaluable patients. Response rates were partial response (27.5%) and stable disease (32.5%). Median time to progression was 20.6 weeks. Median overall survival was 36 weeks. Major hematologic toxicity included grade 3 anemia 4.3%, neutropenia 1.7%, and thrombocytopenia 2.38%. In addition, reported grade II toxicity included neuropathy 7.5%, ototoxicity 7.5%, rash 7.14%, and nausea and vomiting 3.5%.

Table 4
Activity of gemcitabine and platinum combinations

Author	N	Gemcitabine	Platinum Compound	Outcome	Comments
Doval et al	30	1000 mg/m2 30–60 min D 1 and 8 Every 3 wk	Cisplatin, 70 mg/m2 D 1 Every 3 wk	RR: 36% TTP: 18 wk OS: 20 wk	Gallbladder cancer patients
Thongprasert et al	43	1250 mg/m2 30 min D 1 and 8 Every 3 wk	Cisplatin, 75 mg/m2 D 1 Every 3 wk	PR: 27.5% TTP: 20 wk OS: 36 wk	Mostly ICC
Lee et al	39	1250 mg/m2 30 min D 1 and 8 Every 3 wk	Cisplatin, 70 mg/m2 D 1 Every 3 wk	PR: 17.1% TTP: 3.2 mon OS: 8.6 mon	—
Julka et al	20	1000 mg/m2 30–60 min D 1 and 8 Every 3 wk	Carboplatin, AUC5 D 1 Every 3 wk	RR: 35.7% OS: 31 wk	Gallbladder cancer patients
Suresh et al	48	1000 mg/m2 30 min D 1 and 8 Every 3 wk	Carboplatin, AUC5 D 1 Every 3 wk	RR: 29.2%	Favorable toxicity profile
Andre et al	33	1000 mg/m2 Fixed dose rate D 1 Every 2 wk	Oxaliplatin, 100 mg/m2 D 2 Every 2 wk	Group A PR: 36% PFS: 5.7 mon OS: 15.4 mon Group B PR: 21.7% PFS: 3.9 mon OS: 7.6 mon	Demonstrates efficacy and safety of palliative chemotherapy in both group A (good PS and normal bilirubin) and group B (poor PS or elevated bilirubin) patients
Harder et al	31	1000 mg/m2 30 min D 1, 8, and 15 Every 4 wk	Oxaliplatin, 100 mg/m2 D 1 and 15 Every 4 wk	PR: 26% TTP: 6.4 mon OS: 11 mon	Febrile neutropenia 7%

Abbreviations: ICC, intra-hepatic cholangiocarcinoma; OS, overall survival; PFS, progression-free survival; PR, partial response; PS, performance status; RR, response rate; TTP, time to progression.

More recently, 39 patients (35 evaluable) with advanced biliary tract cancer were treated with cisplatin, 70 mg/m^2 day 1, followed by gemcitabine, 1250 mg/m^2 days 1 and 8, repeated every 3 weeks for a maximum of eight cycles.[24] Intrahepatic cholangiocarcinoma represented 51.4% of cases, and gallbladder cancer represented 40% of cases. The response rates were 17.1% partial response and 28.6% stable disease. Median time to progression was 3.2 months. Median overall survival was 8.6 months. Toxicity was reported per cycle administered (N = 148). Grade 3 and 4 adverse events of cycles administered included neutropenia 35.8%, thrombocytopenia 17.6%, anemia 6.8%, nausea 3.4%, vomiting 2.7%, constipation 2%, and febrile neutropenia 1.4%.

The combination of gemcitabine and carboplatin was tested in a phase II study that enrolled 20 patients with advanced gallbladder cancer.[25] Carboplatin was selected given its better toxicity profile in terms of nephropathy and neuropathy when compared with cisplatin. Treatment plan included gemcitabine, 1000 mg/m^2 30- to 60-minute IV infusion days 1 and 8, followed by carboplatin AUC5, 45- to 60-minute IV infusion on day 1 of an every 3-week cycle for a maximum of six cycles. Reported response rates were complete response 20%, partial response 15.7%, and stable disease 31.5%. Median overall survival was 31.7 weeks and 1-year overall survival was 43.3%. Grade 3 and 4 toxicities included anemia 15%, neutropenia 10%, and thrombocytopenia 5%. Grade 1 and 2 nausea and vomiting were observed in 25% of patients and there were no cases of febrile neutropenia.

In a second study, 48 eligible patients with advanced biliary tract cancer were treated with gemcitabine at 1000 mg/m^2 IV over 30 minutes on days 1 and 8 with carboplatin at AUC5 IV on day 1 of a 21-day cycle.[26] Complete and partial responses were reported in 14 patients (29.2%), and stable disease was reported in 24 (50%). Grade 3 hematologic toxicity included neutropenia 33%, febrile neutropenia 0.02%, anemia 12.5%, and thrombocytopenia 14.6%. Rates of grade 4 hematologic toxicities were rare neutropenia 0.04% and thrombocytopenia 0.06%. Grade 3 nonhematologic toxicities occurred in three patients and grade 4 depression occurred in one patient. Authors concluded that this combination is active against biliary cancer and is highly tolerable.

The activity of oxaliplatin has also been examined in combination with gemcitabine. In a phase II study, patients with advanced biliary tract cancer were grouped according to performance status and serum bilirubin.[27] Thirty-three patients were included in group A (performance status 0–2 and bilirubin <2.5 times normal) and 23 patients were included in group B (performance status >2, bilirubin >2.5 times normal or prior chemotherapy). Patients were treated with gemcitabine, 1000 mg/m^2 fixed dose rate day 1, and oxaliplatin, 100 mg/m^2 day 2, every 2 weeks. Efficacy results were reported separately. For group A patients, response rates were partial response 36% and stable disease 26%. Median progression-free survival was 5.7 months and median overall survival 15.4 months. For group B patients, response rates were complete response 4.3%, partial response 17.4%, and stable disease 30%. Median progression-free survival was 3.9 months and median overall survival 7.6 months. Grade 3 and 4 toxicities were reported for all 56 patients together and included neutropenia 14%, anemia 9%, thrombocytopenia 9%, nausea and vomiting 5.3%, and neuropathy 7.1%. Authors emphasized differences in prognostic factors as a reason for the wide spectrum of results reported in phase II trials and concluded that this combination is active and well tolerated even in the subgroup of patients with poor prognostic factors.

A slightly different schedule was tested in a second phase II trial of the gemcitabine and oxaliplatin combination. Thirty-one patients with advanced biliary tract cancer were treated with gemcitabine, 1000 mg/m^2 30-minute IV infusion days 1, 8, and 15, and oxaliplatin, 100 mg/m^2 days 1 and 15, of an every 4-week cycle.[28] Reported response rates were partial response 26% and stable disease 45%. Median time to progression was 6.4 months and median overall survival 11 months. Grade 3 and 4 toxicities included thrombocytopenia 23%, neuropathy 19%, leukocytopenia 16%, anemia 10%, and febrile neutropenia 7%. Authors concluded that their results confirmed the activity of the combination in patients with advanced biliary tract cancer.

Gemcitabine and Fluoropyrimidine Combinations

The combination of gemcitabine and fluoropyrimidines (**Table 5**) was selected for patients with biliary tract cancer given the single-agent activity of both drugs, possible synergistic activity, and nonoverlapping toxicity profile. Preliminary evidence of the activity of the combination of gemcitabine and infusional 5-fluorouracil came from a retrospective review of the experience of a single institution. At the Princess Margaret Hospital, 27 patients were treated with gemcitabine at 900 mg/m^2 days 1, 8, and 15 every 4 weeks, plus 5-fluorouracil continuous infusion at 200 mg/m^2/d for 21 days every 4 weeks.[29] ECOG 2 and 3 patients represented 56% of the cases. Objective responses were noted in 33% of the patients and stable disease was observed in 30% of the patients. Median overall survival was 5.1 months. Grade 3 and 4 toxicities included line infection 19%, mucositis 11%, deep venous thrombosis 11%, neutropenia 7%, fatigue 7%, diarrhea 4%, nausea 4%, thrombocytopenia 4%, and febrile neutropenia 4%. Authors concluded that the combination was active, but the toxicity had to be minimized. Of note, half of the serious adverse events in this report were related to catheter complications. These results could not be replicated when gemcitabine was combined with bolus 5-fluorouracil. Forty-two patients with advanced biliary tract cancer were included in a phase II trial.[30] The regimen consisted of gemcitabine, 1000 mg/m^2 30-minute IV infusion days 1, 8, and 15; leucovorin, 25 mg/m^2 IV bolus; and 5-fluorouracil, 600 mg/m^2 IV bolus in an every 4-week cycle. A partial response was observed in 12% of patients, median time to progression was 4.6 months, and median overall survival was 9.7 months. Grade 3 adverse events included neutropenia 40.6%, thrombocytopenia 18.8%, nausea 12.5%, vomiting 12.5%, thrombosis 9.45%, fatigue 21.9%, infection without neutropenia 9.4%, and infection with neutropenia 3.1%. Grade 4 adverse events included neutropenia 18.8%, thrombosis 6.3%, and leucopenia 3.1%. The authors concluded that response rates and survival were equivalent to those reported for single-agent gemcitabine.

A formal phase II evaluation of the combination of gemcitabine and capecitabine was conducted with the expectation that results observed with infusional 5-fluorouracil could be reproduced without the associated catheter-related complications.[31] Forty-five patients with advanced biliary tract cancer were treated with gemcitabine, 1000 mg/m^2 30-minute IV infusion days 1 and 8, plus capecitabine, 650 mg/m^2 orally twice a day for 14 days in a 3-week cycle. ECOG performance status of 0 or 1 was observed in 82% of the patients. Response rates were complete response 4%, partial response 27%, and stable disease 42%. Median progression-free survival was 7 months and median overall survival was 14 months. Grade 3 toxicity included neutropenia 32%, thrombocytopenia 11%, hand-foot rash 9%, infection 4%, fatigue 4%, and febrile neutropenia 2%. The authors noticed that the toxicity profile was similar even for patients with serum bilirubin 1.5 to 3 times the upper limit of normal, a common clinical scenario in patients with advanced biliary tract cancer. It was concluded that this regimen was active and well tolerated. The authors recommended that the gemcitabine and capecitabine combination should be evaluated in a phase III

Table 5
Gemcitabine and fluoropyrimidine combinations

Author	N	Gemcitabine	Fluoropyrimidine	Outcome	Comments
Alberts et al	42	1000 mg/m2 30 min D 1, 8, and 15 Every 4 wk	LV, 25 mg/m2 bolus and 5-FU, 600 mg/ m2 bolus D 1, 8, and 15 Every 4 wk	PR: 12% TTP: 4.6 mon OS: 9.7 mon	Outcome similar to single-agent gemcitabine.
Knox et al	45	1000 mg/m2 30 min D 1 and 8 Every 3 wk	Capecitabine, 650 mg/m2 twice a day D 1–14 Every 3 wk	RR: 31% PFS: 7 mon OS: 14 mon	Active and well tolerated regimen. Febrile neutropenia 2%.
Cho et al	44	1000 mg/m2 30 min D 1 and 8 Every 3 wk	Capecitabine, 650 mg/m2 twice a day D 1–14 Every 3 wk	PR: 32% TTP: 6 mon OS: 14 mon	Active and well tolerated. Febrile neutropenia 6%.
Iyer et al	12	1000 mg/m2 30 min D 1 and 8 Every 3 wk	Capecitabine, 650 mg/m2 twice a day D 1–14 Every 3 wk	PR: 2/12 TTP: 9 mon OS: 14 mon	Suggests maintained quality of life.

Abbreviations: 5-FU, 5-fluorouracil; LV, leucovorin; OS, overall survival; PFS, progression-free survival; PR, partial response; RR, response rate; TTP, time to progression.

trial in advanced disease and in the adjuvant setting. Similar results have been obtained in two additional phase II studies conducted in Korea[32] and the United States.[33]

Targeted Agents

Recently, preclinical studies have highlighted the relevance of endothelial growth factor receptor, the MAPK pathway, and angiogenesis in the pathogenesis of biliary tract cancers. Accordingly, the activity of targeted agents has been examined in patients with advanced biliary tract cancer. Erlotinib, an endothelial growth factor receptor tyrosine kinase inhibitor, was evaluated in a phase II trial that included 42 patients.[34] Of note, endothelial growth factor receptor–HER1 expression by immunohistochemistry was positive in 81% of the patients and 57% of patients had been treated with systemic chemotherapy previously. Patients received erlotinib, 150 mg/day orally continuously. Response rates were partial response 8% and stable disease 43%. Median duration of the stable disease was 4.4 months. The 6-month progression-free survival was 17%, median time to progression 2.6 months, and the median overall survival 7.5 months. Grade 3 toxicities included vomiting 7.1%, skin rash 4.7%, nausea 4.7%, fatigue 2.3%, bilirubin 2.3%, aspartate aminotransferase 2.3%, and hyponatremia 2.3%. Most frequent grade 1 and 2 toxicities were skin rash 73.8%, fatigue 50%, and diarrhea 40.4%. One of three of the patients who experienced a partial response did not express endothelial growth factor receptor by immunohistochemistry. Although the predefined threshold to declare activity of erlotinib in this disease was not met (progression-free survival 20% at 6 months), the authors emphasized the inclusion of a mixed population of patients regarding previous systemic therapy and concluded that erlotinib may offer a therapeutic option after failure to systemic chemotherapy given that 5 (20.8%) of 24 patients with advanced biliary tract cancer who received erlotinib in the second-line setting were progression free at 6 months.

Sorafenib, an oral multikinase inhibitor, blocks tumor cell proliferation by targeting Raf/MEK/ERK signaling at the level of Raf kinase, and exerts an antiangiogenic effect by targeting vascular endothelial growth factor receptor-2 and -3, and platelet-derived growth factor receptor-β tyrosine kinases.[35] Thirty-six patients with advanced biliary tract cancer and no prior systemic treatment received sorafenib, 400 mg orally twice a day continuously in a phase II trial.[36] In terms of efficacy, response rates were partial response 6% and stable disease 29%. Median progression-free survival was 2 months and median overall survival was 6 months. Grade 3 and 4 toxicities occurred in 66.7% of patients and included hand-foot syndrome 13%, thromboembolism 10%, elevated liver enzymes 10%, and abdominal pain 10%. Reversible posterior leukoencephalopathy syndrome, gastrointestinal perforation, and gastrointestinal hemorrhage were each seen in 3% of patients. One patient died with grade 4 supraventricular tachycardia and venous thromboembolism. Authors concluded that although response rates were low, survival was comparable with that attributed to commonly used chemotherapy regimens. Sorafenib is currently under testing with combination chemotherapy in biliary tract cancers.

REGIONAL CHEMOTHERAPY FOR ADVANCED DISEASE

At Memorial Sloan-Kettering Cancer Center, 26 patients with unresectable intrahepatic cholangiocarcinoma with disease confined to the liver were treated with hepatic arterial infusion of floxuridine at 0.16 mg/kg/d and dexamethasone from days 1 to 14 followed by heparinized saline from days 15 to 28. Cycles were repeated every 28 days. Response rates were partial response 54% and stable disease 42%. Median disease-specific survival was 31 months. One patient's disease was rendered resectable and a pathologic complete response was documented. Three grade 3 complications (bilirubin, pain, gastrointestinal) and two grade 4 complications (bilirubin) were reported.[37] These results compare favorably with those of 18 patients with intrahepatic cholangiocarcinoma treated with capecitabine and oxaliplatin where no objective responses were observed and median survival was 5.2 months.

ADJUVANT CHEMOTHERAPY

The role of adjuvant chemotherapy after resection of pancreatobiliary malignancies has been investigated in Japan, where a large multi-institutional phase III trial was conducted.[38] Stage II to IV resected patients were randomized to adjuvant chemotherapy or observation. Chemotherapy consisted of mitomycin-C, 6 mg/m^2 the day of surgery, followed by a slow IV infusion of 5-flurouracil, 310 mg/m^2 for 5 consecutive days on weeks 1 and 3 after surgery, followed by daily oral 5-fluorouracil, 100 mg/m^2 until progression of disease. The primary end point was overall survival. Patients were also monitored for disease-recurrence and underwent monthly assessments with physical examination, laboratory studies, radiographs, ultrasound, and CT scans. All patients were followed for 5 years. The trial attempted stratification by primary site (gallbladder, pancreatic, biliary, ampullary carcinoma) and the hypothesis was that systemic chemotherapy could improve 5-year survival from 15% to 35% for each subgroup of patients. A total of 508 patients were enrolled and randomly allocated to postoperative chemotherapy or observation. Of interest for this article, the study randomized 139 bile duct carcinoma patients and 140 gallbladder carcinoma patients. When all 508 patients were analyzed, there was a statistically significant advantage in terms of overall survival that favored patients who had received chemotherapy. The 5-year survival rate was 14.4% for the control group and 26% for the chemotherapy group ($P = .0367$). The 5-year survival rate of gallbladder carcinoma patients was significantly better in the chemotherapy group (26%) compared with the control group (14.4%) ($P = .0367$, two-sided log-rank test). The benefit of adjuvant chemotherapy seemed to be restricted to those patients with gallbladder carcinoma who had undergone a noncurative resection. In this setting, the 5-year survival rate was 8.9% in the chemotherapy group and 0% in the control group ($P = .0226$). Of note, the intention-to-treat analysis did not reveal differences in terms of overall survival or disease-free survival and this was attributed to an imbalance in the number of ineligible patients caused by stage I disease: 3 patients in the chemotherapy group and 20 patients in the control group. The 5-year survival of patients with bile duct carcinoma was not different in the chemotherapy group (26.7%) when compared with the control group (24.1%).

No other randomized trials examining the efficacy of systemic chemotherapy in patients with resectable biliary tract cancer in the adjuvant or neoadjuvant setting were identified. The anecdotal report of significant downstaging of an initially unresectable intrahepatic cholangiocarcinoma in a patient treated with regional chemotherapy reported previously is the only light on a possibly promising neoadjuvant approach, which may deserve further evaluation.

Two current studies evaluating systemic chemotherapy in the adjuvant setting are underway. One is evaluating the combination of gemcitabine plus oxaliplatin, and the other single-agent gemcitabine.

SUMMARY

Advanced biliary tract carcinomas represent a group of aggressive diseases with an associated poor prognosis. In selected patients, chemotherapy has the potential for providing symptom control and may also prolong survival. Combination chemotherapy seems to be more effective than single-agent chemotherapy in the palliative setting but confirmation from phase III trials that include quality of life as an end point are awaited. The reference chemotherapy regimen for advanced disease has not been identified but arguably is either gemcitabine or fluoropyrimidine base. Medical oncologists need to individualize the selection according to the patient characteristics and associated comorbidities. A gemcitabine and cisplatin regimen seems appropriate in patients with good performance. Targeted therapies have shown limited activity and further research is needed to understand better their role in this disease. Potential combination with chemotherapy may help improve their effect and is to be further studied. For those patients with completely resected disease, there is no role for adjuvant chemotherapy and phase III trials evaluating most active combinations are urgently needed.

REFERENCES

1. Ries LAG, Melbert D, Krapcho M, et al, editors. SEER cancer statistics review. Bethesda (MD): National Cancer Institute; 2005.
2. Patel T. Increasing incidence and mortality of primary intrahepatic cholangiocarcinoma in the United States. Hepatology 2001;33(6):1353–7.
3. Jemal A, Siegel R, Ward E, et al. Cancer statistics, 2008. CA Cancer J Clin 2008; 58(2):71–96.
4. Jarnagin WR, Ruo L, Little SA, et al. Patterns of initial disease recurrence after resection of gallbladder carcinoma and hilar cholangiocarcinoma: implications for adjuvant therapeutic strategies. Cancer 2003;98(8):1689–700.
5. Fong Y, Blumgart LH, Lin E, et al. Outcome of treatment for distal bile duct cancer. Br J Surg 1996;83(12):1712–5.
6. Endo I, Gonen M, Yopp AC, et al. Intrahepatic cholangiocarcinoma: rising frequency, improved survival, and determinants of outcome after resection. Ann Surg 2008;248(1):84–96.
7. Eckel F, Schmid RM. Chemotherapy in advanced biliary tract carcinoma: a pooled analysis of clinical trials. Br J Cancer 2007;96(6):896–902.
8. Jarnagin WR, Klimstra DS, Hezel M, et al. Differential cell cycle-regulatory protein expression in biliary tract adenocarcinoma: correlation with anatomic site, pathologic variables, and clinical outcome. J Clin Oncol 2006;24(7):1152–60.
9. Glimelius B, Hoffman K, Sjoden PO, et al. Chemotherapy improves survival and quality of life in advanced pancreatic and biliary cancer. Ann Oncol 1996;7(6):593–600.
10. Ducreux M, Van Cutsem E, Van Laethem JL, et al. A randomised phase II trial of weekly high-dose 5-fluorouracil with and without folinic acid and cisplatin in patients with advanced biliary tract carcinoma: results of the 40955 EORTC trial. Eur J Cancer 2005;41(3):398–403.
11. Valle JW, Wasan H, Johnson P, et al. Gemcitabine, alone or in combination with cisplatin, in patients with advanced or metastatic cholangiocarcinomas and other biliary tract tumors: a multicentre randomised phase II study. In 2006 Gastrointestinal Cancers Symposium. San Francisco (CA) 2006.
12. Kornek GV, Schuell B, Laengle F, et al. Mitomycin C in combination with capecitabine or biweekly high-dose gemcitabine in patients with advanced biliary tract cancer: a randomised phase II trial. Ann Oncol 2004;15(3):478–83.
13. Rao S, Cunningham D, Hawkins RE, et al. Phase III study of 5FU, etoposide and leucovorin (FELV) compared to epirubicin, cisplatin and 5FU (ECF) in previously untreated patients with advanced biliary cancer. Br J Cancer 2005;92(9):1650–4.

14. Ducreux M, Rougier P, Fandi A, et al. Effective treatment of advanced biliary tract carcinoma using 5-fluorouracil continuous infusion with cisplatin. Ann Oncol 1998;9(6):653–6.

15. Taieb J, Mitry E, Boige V, et al. Optimization of 5-fluorouracil (5-FU)/cisplatin combination chemotherapy with a new schedule of leucovorin, 5-FU and cisplatin (LV5FU2-P regimen) in patients with biliary tract carcinoma. Ann Oncol 2002;13(8):1192–6.

16. Sanz-Altamira PM, Ferrante K, Jenkins RL, et al. A phase II trial of 5-fluorouracil, leucovorin, and carboplatin in patients with unresectable biliary tree carcinoma. Cancer 1998;82(12):2321–5.

17. Nehls O, Klump B, Arkenau HT, et al. Oxaliplatin, fluorouracil and leucovorin for advanced biliary system adenocarcinomas: a prospective phase II trial. Br J Cancer 2002;87(7):702–4.

18. Lim JY, Jeung HC, Mun HS, et al. Phase II trial of oxaliplatin combined with leucovorin and fluorouracil for recurrent/metastatic biliary tract carcinoma. Anticancer Drugs 2008;19(6):631–5.

19. Nehls O, Oettle H, Hartmann JT, et al. Capecitabine plus oxaliplatin as first-line treatment in patients with advanced biliary system adenocarcinoma: a prospective multicentre phase II trial. Br J Cancer 2008;98(2):309–15.

20. Carraro S, Servienti PJ, Bruno MF, et al. Gemcitabine and cisplatin in locally advanced or metastatic gallbladder and bile duct adenocarcinomas. Proc Am Soc Clin Oncol 2001;20 [abstract 2333].

21. Malik IA, Aziz Z, Zaidi SH, et al. Gemcitabine and cisplatin is a highly effective combination chemotherapy in patients with advanced cancer of the gallbladder. Am J Clin Oncol 2003;26(2):174–7.

22. Doval DC, Sekhon JS, Gupta SK, et al. A phase II study of gemcitabine and cisplatin in chemotherapy-naive, unresectable gall bladder cancer. Br J Cancer 2004;90(8):1516–20.

23. Thongprasert S, Napapan S, Charoentum C, et al. Phase II study of gemcitabine and cisplatin as first-line chemotherapy in inoperable biliary tract carcinoma. Ann Oncol 2005;16(2):279–81.

24. Lee J, Kim TY, Lee MA, et al. Phase II trial of gemcitabine combined with cisplatin in patients with inoperable biliary tract carcinomas. Cancer Chemother Pharmacol 2008;61(1):47–52.

25. Julka PK, Puri T, Rath GK. A phase II study of gemcitabine and carboplatin combination chemotherapy in gallbladder carcinoma. Hepatobiliary Pancreat Dis Int 2006;5(1):110–4.

26. Suresh R, Picus J, Sorscher S, et al. Gemcitabine and carboplatin in the treatment of metastatic cholangiocarcinoma and gallbladder cancer. 2007 ASCO Annual Meeting Proceedings Part I. J Clin Oncol 2007;25(18S). (June 20 Supplement) [abstract 15102].

27. Andre T, Tournigand C, Rosmorduc O, et al. Gemcitabine combined with oxaliplatin (GEMOX) in advanced biliary tract adenocarcinoma: a GERCOR study. Ann Oncol 2004;15(9):1339–43.

28. Harder J, Riecken B, Kummer O, et al. Outpatient chemotherapy with gemcitabine and oxaliplatin in patients with biliary tract cancer. Br J Cancer 2006;95(7):848–52.

29. Knox JJ, Hedley D, Oza A, et al. Gemcitabine concurrent with continuous infusional 5-fluorouracil in advanced biliary cancers: a review of the Princess Margaret Hospital experience. Ann Oncol 2004;15(5):770–4.

30. Alberts SR, Al-Khatib H, Mahoney MR, et al. Gemcitabine, 5-fluorouracil, and leu-covorin in advanced biliary tract and gallbladder carcinoma: a North Central Cancer Treatment Group phase II trial. Cancer 2005;103(1):111–8.
31. Knox JJ, Hedley D, Oza A, et al. Combining gemcitabine and capecitabine in patients with advanced biliary cancer: a phase II trial. J Clin Oncol 2005; 23(10):2332–8.
32. Cho JY, Paik YH, Chang YS, et al. Capecitabine combined with gemcitabine (CapGem) as first-line treatment in patients with advanced/metastatic biliary tract carcinoma. Cancer 2005;104(12):2753–8.
33. Iyer RV, Gibbs J, Kuvshinoff B, et al. A phase II study of gemcitabine and cape-citabine in advanced cholangiocarcinoma and carcinoma of the gallbladder: a single-institution prospective study. Ann Surg Oncol 2007;14(11):3202–9.
34. Philip PA, Mahoney MR, Allmer C, et al. Phase II study of erlotinib in patients with advanced biliary cancer. J Clin Oncol 2006;24(19):3069–74.
35. Wilhelm SM, Carter C, Tang L, et al. BAY 43-9006 exhibits broad spectrum oral antitumor activity and targets the RAF/MEK/ERK pathway and receptor tyrosine kinases involved in tumor progression and angiogenesis. Cancer Res 2004; 64(19):7099–109.
36. El-Khoueiry AB, Rankin C, Lenz HJ, et al. SWOG 0514: a phase II study of sora-fenib (BAY 43-9006) as single agent in patients (pts) with unresectable or meta-static gallbladder cancer or cholangiocarcinomas. 2007 ASCO Annual Meeting Proceedings Part I. J Clin Oncol 2007;25(18S) [abstract 4639].
37. Jarnagin WR, Schwartz LH, Gultekin DH, et al. Hepatic arterial infusional (HAI) therapy in patients with unresectable primary liver cancer: use of dynamic contrast enhanced MRI to evaluate response. J Clin Oncol 2008;26(Suppl) [abstract 4597].
38. Takada T, Amano H, Yasuda H, et al. Is postoperative adjuvant chemotherapy useful for gallbladder carcinoma? A phase III multicenter prospective random-ized controlled trial in patients with resected pancreaticobiliary carcinoma. Cancer 2002;95(8):1685–95.

Index

Note: Page numbers of article titles are in **boldface** type.

A

Adjuvant therapy, after surgery for gallbladder cancer, 317–318
    percutaneous, for biliary malignancies, 248–251
        portal vein embolization, 249–251
        transcatheter chemoembolization and radioembolization, 248–249
    with surgery for intrahepatic cholangiocarcinoma, 298–299
Anatomy, in biliary tract malignancies, 241–242, 243–244

B

Benign biliary stricture, dilemmas in diagnosis of, **207–214**
    causes of, 211–212
    definition, 207–208
    radiographic evaluation of, 208–211
    serologic studies, 208
    tissue sampling, 211
Beta-Catenin, role in cholangiocarcinogenesis, 219
Bile duct, intraductal papillary neoplasm of, as precursor to cholangiocarcinoma, **215–224**
Bile duct resection, for gallbladder cancer, 316
Biliary cystadenocarcinoma. *See* Cystadenocarcinoma, biliary.
Biliary drainage. *See* Drainage, biliary.
Biliary intraepithelial neoplasia, as precursor to cholangiocarcinoma, **215–224**
Biliary malignancies, 207–375
    cholangiocarcinogenesis, **215–224**
        biliary intraepithelial neoplasia, 216
        cell cycle proteins, 217
        cell-adhesion proteins, 219
        intraductal papillary neoplasm of bile duct, 216
        matrix proteins, 220
        mucinous proteins, 218–219
        tumor suppressor genes, 217–218
    diagnosis of nonmalignant biliary obstruction *versus*, **207–214**
        causes of benign biliary stricture, 211–212
        definition, 207–208
        radiographic evaluation of, 208–211
        serologic studies, 208
        tissue sampling, 211
    extrahepatic cholangiocarcinoma, **267–286**
        classification, 267–268
        palliative management, 279
        patterns of failure, 279
        prognostic factors after surgical treatment, 275–278

Surg Oncol Clin N Am 18 (2009) 381–391
doi:10.1016/S1055-3207(09)00009-X
1055-3207/09/$ – see front matter © 2009 Elsevier Inc. All rights reserved.

surgonc.theclinics.com

388 Index

Moving?

Make sure your subscription moves with you!

To notify us of your new address, find your **Clinics Account Number** (located on your mailing label above your name), and contact customer service at:

E-mail: elspcs@elsevier.com

800-654-2452 (subscribers in the U.S. & Canada)
314-453-7041 (subscribers outside of the U.S. & Canada)

Fax number: 314-523-5170

Elsevier Periodicals Customer Service
11830 Westline Industrial Drive
St. Louis, MO 63146

*To ensure uninterrupted delivery of your subscription, please notify us at least 4 weeks in advance of move.

Printed and bound by CPI Group (UK) Ltd, Croydon, CR0 4YY

03/10/2024

01040453-0019